Self-Development Outweighs Sheer Skill

Yoga is the oldest known science of self-development. It is mental, physical and spiritual control. *Yoga for Every Athlete* is the result of more than 20 years of experimentation and experience in the application of yoga in sports. Here you will find guidelines on using yoga for mental and physical preparation and strength regeneration from olympic coach and sports psychologist Dr. Aladar Kogler. Using examples of his top athletes, Dr. Kogler illustrates how yoga conditions the body for optimal sports training and how you can tailor a program that meets your personal goals and needs. *Yoga for Every Athlete* contains 27 exercise batteries for virtually any sport in which you participate: be it bicycling, golf, running, fencing—your performance level and enjoyment will radically improve with only 10 minutes of Yoga practice a day.

No matter what condition your body is in, Dr. Kogler's methods will increase your strength, agility, outlook, body shape and overall mental, emotional and physical health. *Yoga For Every Athlete* is based on the fact that bodily processes, such as heart rate and blood flow, can be influenced by your will. This means that your peak physical performance actually lies in your own mental preparation.

Learning and practicing Yoga feels good because it positively affects both mind and body. When you practice Yoga you simultaneously complete several training tasks at one time, resulting in the most efficient use of training time and energy.

ABOUT THE AUTHOR

Aladar Kogler, Ph.D is co-head coach of the Columbia University's men's and women's fencing teams in New York City. He is also the director of the Sport Psychology Laboratory at Columbia University, established in 1984 by the United States Olympic Committee and Columbia University for the United States Fencing Association Sport Medicine Program.

A native of Hungary, Kogler holds a Master of Fencing Degree from the Hungarian College of Higher Physical Education in Budapest, a master and doctorate degree from two Czechoslovakian universities—Comenius University in Bratislava and Carl University in Prague. In addition, he earned the scientific post doctoral degree in Eastern Europe—the Candidate of Science (CSc). In 1974, the Czechoslovak government awarded him its highest award for coaching. He was professor at Comenius University and the head olympic coach for the Czechoslovak fencing team until 1981 when he emigrated to the United States. Here, he lead the Wayne State University's men's fencing team to the 1982-83 NCAA Champion title and the women's team to the runner-up title. He has been named co-technical director of the U.S. Olympic Sport Medicine Program for fencing, and consultant for the U.S. Olympic Sport Science Committee. He is the weapon coordinator for the men's epee fencing in the USFA.

Since 1983 he has been with Columbia University. During his time there, the fencing team won five NCAA Championships, three men's titles and two combined men's and women's titles. He has coached fourteen individual NCAA champions in several weapons, eighteen national champions, pan american champions, world cup and World University Games finalists. He was the U.S. Olympic coach for both the Seoul and Barcelona Fencing teams and three-time U.S. Pan American coach.

TO WRITE THE AUTHOR

If you wish to contact the author, please write to him or her in care of Llewellyn Worldwide, and we will forward your letter. Both the author and the publisher appreciate hearing from you and learning of your enjoyment of this book and how it has helped you. Llewellyn Worldwide cannot guarantee that every letter written to the author can be answered, but all will be forwarded. Please write to:

Aladar Kogler, Ph.D.

c/o Llewellyn Worldwide

P.O. Box 64383-K387, St. Paul, MN 55164-0383, U.S.A.

Please enclose a self-addressed, stamped envelope or $1.00 to cover costs.
If outside the U.S.A., enclose international postal reply coupon.

LLEWELLYN'S STRATEGIES FOR SUCCESS SERIES

YOGA

FOR

EVERY ATHLETE

SECRETS OF AN OLYMPIC COACH

ALADAR KOGLER, PH.D.
SPORTS PSYCHOLOGIST

1995
LLEWELLYN PUBLICATIONS
ST. PAUL, MINNESOTA 55164-0383 U.S.A.

FIRST EDITION
Second Printing, 1995

Center cover image by Katherine Lane
Other cover photos ©1995 PhotoDisc, Inc.
Cover design by Lynne Menturweck
Interior photos by Katherine Lane
Interior design, layout and editing by Laura Gudbaur
Models for interior photographs: Sharon Monplasir, member of the 1984, 1988, 1992 U.S. Olympic Fencing Team; Michael Gostigian, member of the 1988 and 1992 U.S. Olympic Modern Pentathalon Team (both trained by the author), Aladar Kogler, Ph.D. (the author)

Library of Congress Cataloging in Publication Data
Kogler, Aladar.
    Yoga for every athlete: secrets of an Olympic coach / Aladar Kogler. -- 1st ed.
        p. cm. -- (Llewellyn's Strategies for Success series)
    Includes bibliographical references and index.
    ISBN 1-56718-387-5 (trade pbk. : alk. paper)
    1. Yoga, Hatha. 2. Yoga, Raja. I. Title. II. Series.
    RA781.7.K644 1995   95-13900
        613.7'046--dc20   CIP

Printed in the United States of America

Llewellyn Publications
A Division of Llewellyn Worldwide Ltd.
St. Paul, Minnesota 55164-0383

ABOUT LLEWELLYN'S
"STRATEGIES FOR SUCCESS" SERIES

The secret to success is really no secret at all. Just ask any successful person. The "secret" is really a universal truth that belongs to each and every human being on the planet. That truth is: Success begins in the mind.

Many of us live from day to day feeling that something is missing, or that we are a victim of circumstances that make success impossible.

The greatest barrier to success is this illusion of helplessness and powerlessness. It is the illusion that you have no choices in life. The successful person knows that this illusion is like a deadly virus to the spirit.

The good news is that you possess the power—*inside yourself now*—to sweep illusions from your mind and begin using your mind for what it was intended: to lift human consciousness to a higher plane and make this planet a better place for yourself and your children.

How is this done?

That's where Llewellyn's "Strategies for Success" come in. Techniques are available that can help you activate your inner resources to create exciting new potentials in your life. These techniques involve intellectual, physical, emotional, as well as psychic improvement.

Yoga concepts and strategies recognize that the source of ultimate power resides within a balance of the mind and body. Combining age-old asanas with mental affirmations, each strategy embodies a firm regard for the divine spark of greatness existing in everyone.

With the techniques presented in this book, you can open the door and enjoy a success beyond your wildest dreams—not only in your athletic performance, but also in your whole life.

Success is your destiny. When you are self-empowered, you become the sole architect of your life. Why wait? Seize your power now.

OTHER BOOKS BY THE AUTHOR

Yoga, Autogenic Training
>Published in Czechoslovakia

Preparing the Mind—Psychological Preparation of Fencers
>Counter Parry Press, PA.

Physical and Mental Preparation of Fencers
>Published in Czechoslovakia

Planning to Win
>Counter Parry Press, PA.

Clearing the Path to Victory: A Self-Guided Mental Training Program for Athletes
>Counter Parry Press, PA.

DEDICATION

I dedicate this book to Selva Raja Jesudian whose book, *Sport Es Joga*, published in Hungary in the 1940s, was my first source of yoga which planted the seed. To Swami Rama, spiritual leader and founder of the Himalayan Institute, whose life, knowledge and works are sources for permanent inspiration. And to Maharishi Mahesh Yogi, founder of Transcendental Meditation.

TABLE OF CONTENTS ━━━

Expansion • The Resting Posture • The Modified Chest Expansion • The Shoulderstand • The Bow • The Seated Forward Bend • The Plough • The Headstand • The Cross-Legged Posture • The Cobra • The Scale • The Fish • The Kneeling Posture • The Abdominal Lift • Nauli • The Relaxation Posture • The Crow • The Side Crow • The Tiptoe Posture • The Triangle "A" • The Triangle with Twist "B" • The Cat Stretch • The Head to Knee Posture • The Shoulder Raise • The "T" Posture • The Body Straight Posture • Padasana Variation "A" • Padasana Variation "B" • Padasana Variation "C" • The Lunge • The Pigeon Posture • The Leg Stretch • The Standing Leg Stretch • Yoga Sit-up • The Half Headstand • The Modified Camel Posture • The Knee Squeeze • The Bridge Posture • Neck Stretch • Summary

PART III: THE REGIMENS

Supplemental Exercise for Athletes • Warm-up Asana Battery • YRE for Short Term Rest • Yoga Battery of Asanas for Cool-down • Asanas to Prevent, Rehabilitate Back Pain • Asanas for Relaxing Tired Legs after Intensive Loading • YRE for Releasing Shoulder Tension • YRE for Releasing Neck Tension • YRE for Rapid Release of Body Tension • YRE for Releasing Tension in the Diaphragm, Abdominal Muscles and to Stimulate and Strengthen the Functions of Digestive Organs • Salutation to the Sun • Salutation to the Moon • Example of Athlete's Total Yoga Training • The "Double R" Breath in Case of High Stress • Rhythimic Yoga Breathing When Walking • The Tension Releasing Breath • Battery of Asanas for Improving Balance and Concentration • Using Yoga as Supplemental Training • Boxing • Biking • Fencing • Golf • Gymnastics (Olympic) • Ice Skating, Ice Hockey, Roller Skating • Shooting, Archery, Yachting, Race Car Driving • Skiing • Swimming, Aquatic Sports • Wrestling and Judo • Weightlifting • Team Sports • Soccer • Tennis, Racquet Sports • Track and Field • Walking, Running • Jumping Events (Long Jump, High Jump, Triple Jump) Throwing Events (Shotput, Javelin, Discus)

Asanas that Activate and Deactivate • Battery of Asanas for Activation (Stimulation) • Battery of Asanas for Deactivation (Calming)

LIST OF ILLUSTRATIONS ▬▬

PREFACE ━━━━━━━

Many factors have affected the birth of this book. One of the main factors was my experience as a teenager and my sport career in Eastern Europe, during the 1950s.

As a child, I lived in the northern part of Hungary. After World War II this area was occupied by Slovak communists, and was annexed into communist Slovakia.

My parents were labeled as Hungarian aristocrats—"capitalists" and "class enemies." In 1949, my brother defected and went to the West.

This may not mean anything special to you, the reader. But those who lived there at that time, know that these "sins" were the biggest ones a person could have committed.

All my parents' property was nationalized and all our personal possessions were seized. Our family was exiled to a small village in the country, which had no electricity or means of communication. We were allowed to take 120 pounds per person from among whatever personal items we had owned.

When my brother defected to the West at age 17, I was expelled from my high school. Later, my father died of a heart attack, and my mother suffered paralysis on the right side of her face.

At age 13, I felt helpless, frustrated, and hopeless.

In order to heal myself and somehow cope, I began searching for and reading books on yoga. At that time, such books were forbidden reading in Eastern Europe. With great earnestness, I studied and practiced yoga. I learned that the yogi draws the power to achieve perfect harmony—inner and outer, physical and mental harmony—from within.

I learned about the remarkable abilities of yogis. They did very unusual and interesting things. Furthermore, they achieved these things by drawing on their own inner power.

I came to realize that my only source of healing and survival was inside of me.

I learned to observe my body and my mind. I learned to control my body. I learned to regulate the movements of my lungs—my breathing. I observed how my thoughts and moods influence my body. I learned about the unity of mind and body. I learned the importance of breath awareness, and through the control of breathing I learned how to calm my mind and how to change my mental states and emotions. I learned how to identify my inner resources (the only resources I could rely on). I learned to control myself.

What I learned from yoga I used not only for my personal healing, but also in my preparation for sport. The techniques that I learned helped me to get to the top in my sport, by giving me an extra edge.

Since I was considered an exceptional young athlete, I put all of my hopes and energy into my sport. As a top athlete, I hoped to survive, to continue my education, to become a world champion and, one day, to be able to defect to the free world.

However, the "final nail in the coffin" of my hopes occurred when I learned that I would not be allowed to compete in any international competitions abroad. I was banned from such competition because my brother had defected to the West. The Slovak police announced to me that if I ever tried to defect, that my younger brother and my mother would face the consequences. Their threats put an end to my athletic career—and to my hopes.

Again, however, I was inspired by yoga to change and to be in control. I devoted myself to studying coaching and teaching. I was determined to train world champions (which I had wanted to be), and to study psychology. I came to see yoga as an ancient form of self-study and self-regulation, and that I could use it in the scientific study of human performance.

Eventually, I received my Ph.D. and CSc (post-doctoral scientific degree). I became a coach and psychologist, and conducted considerable research.

I also became the coach of the Czechoslovakian National Fencing Team. I was the Czechoslovak Olympic Fencing coach, producing world class fencers.

In 1981, after the Moscow Olympics, I defected to the United States. Here, I soon became a U.S. National, Pan American and Olympic coach. All of those personal and professional experiences have played a role in the contents of this book.

Another important factor in the book has been my athletes. Both as coach and psychologist, I have guided athletes from the beginner level (age 9-10) to the world championship level. I've learned a lot from them during the last 30 years. Their successes, both here and in Eastern Europe, have given me (and them) a strong belief in the effectiveness of yoga self-regulation.

During my past 10 years in the United States, I have produced 18 individual national fencing champions; 12 individual NCAA champions in different weapons; a number of Olympians for the Olympic games in Los Angeles, Seoul, and Barcelona; Pan-American Gold Medalists; a number of World Cup finalists; World University Game Finalists, Pan American finalists; and coached 5 NCAA championship teams.

I do not exaggerate when I say that the mental preparation based on yoga techniques of my athletes has given me an extra advantage, so that we could compete successfully with countries and coaches who had far superior conditions. My early recognition of the role played by self-regulation (which I was forced to seek and which I did not yet understand), gave me the extra advantage.

I believe that my achievements as a coach/psychologist are 60to 70 percent due to my coaching ability, and 30 to 40 percent due to yoga preparation and self-regulation. I literally believe that my learning of yoga self-regulation techniques saved my life and my career. I learned them, taught them, and then re-learned them again, from the many athletes with whom I worked.

Aladar Kogler, Ph.D.

INTRODUCTION
CHOOSING A DAILY YOGA
EXERCISE PROGRAM

This book offers a holistic training approach for athletes, unifying body and mind through yoga. Many yoga exercises and techniques derived from yoga practice are presented as a way of achieving greater synthesis of body and mind and increased ability for rejuvenating the body. I suggest reading the entire book before beginning the exercises.

Sports training requires a holistic approach. The human being is a psychosomatic unit. There is no mind-body separation. The mind influences the body and vice versa. Athletes are no exception to this rule. A holistic approach is required both when aiming for top competitive results

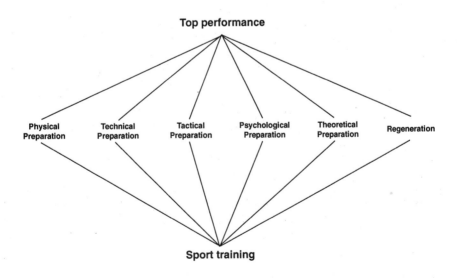

Table 1: Holistic Approach to Training

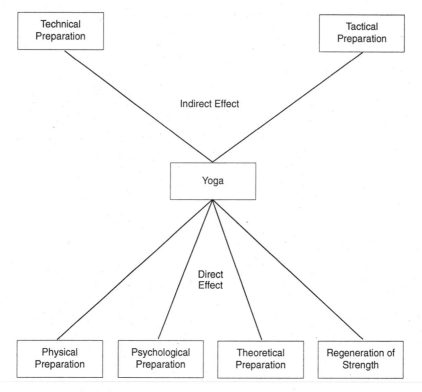

Table 2: The Effect of Yoga on Sport Preparation

as well as when seeking a greater sense of well being and deeper unity of body, mind, and spirit. As Table 1 indicates, physical, technical, tactical, theoretical, and psychological preparation and regeneration (recovery) are inseparable units.

Yoga exercises and techniques derived from yoga indirectly affect technical and tactical preparation. Yoga exercises and techniques also have significant, direct effects on the physical, psychological, theoretical preparation and on the regeneration of the strength process (Table 2).

Yoga asanas can be used for warm-up, cool-down, regeneration, compensation of muscle dysbalances, synthesis of mind and body, activation or deactivation of the body, and as supplemental exercises (Table 3).

Psychological preparation can be divided into two types: general and specific. The task of general psychological preparation is to develop basic mental skills such as goal setting, relaxation techniques, concentration, and visualization (useful also for non-athletes seeking general well-being and a deeper mind-body-spirit union) (Table 4).

Specific psychological preparation readies the athlete for the upcoming competition. The ultimate goal of psychological preparation is self-mastery: control of emotions and control of the mind. This goal is achieved through several steps. (See Table 5 and Table 6)

In order to control your body and mind, you must first understand them. Self-knowledge is gained through self-study and self-observation. You must learn to listen to your body, learn your own body language, and understand your mind and how it works.

The four necessary basic steps towards self-mastery are: body awareness (body control) breath awareness (breath control), attention focus (self-discipline), and concentration. Through these steps and exercises you will learn to listen to your body, become familiar with your body language, and understand how your mind works. You will learn body awareness, how to control and to still your body, breath awareness, and how to control your breath. You will become aware of how to control your mind. You will experience the remarkable benefits of yoga that come from knowing yourself and from knowing that you have the ability to control your autonomic, or unconscious, functions.

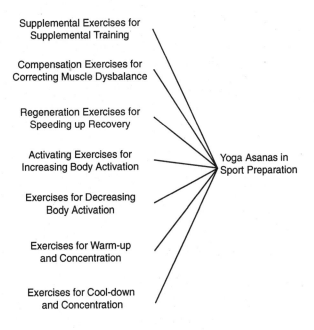

Supplemental Exercises for
Supplemental Training

Compensation Exercises for
Correcting Muscle Dysbalance

Regeneration Exercises for
Speeding up Recovery

Activating Exercises for
Increasing Body Activation

Exercises for Decreasing
Body Activation

Exercises for Warm-up
and Concentration

Exercises for Cool-down
and Concentration

Yoga Asanas in
Sport Preparation

Table 3: Yoga Asanas in Sport Preparation

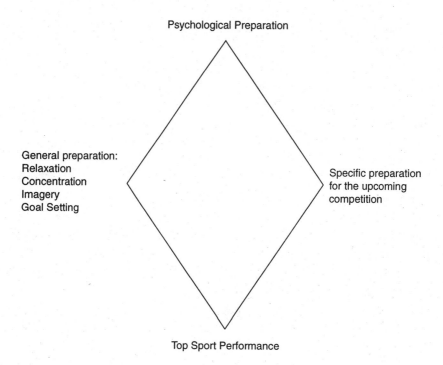

Psychological Preparation

General preparation:
Relaxation
Concentration
Imagery
Goal Setting

Specific preparation
for the upcoming
competition

Top Sport Performance

Table 4: The Tasks of Psychological Preparation

The necessary exercises for daily practice include (Table 5):
Step 1: Body Awareness (Control)

- Sitting still steadily (calming the body)
- Small battery of yoga asanas

Step 2: Breath Awareness (Control)

- Diaphragmatic (abdominal) breathing
  Natural, deep, smooth, even rhythmic breathing
- Complete yoga breathing
- Alternate nostril breathing
- The double "R" breath

Step 3: Attention Focus

- Breath awareness focus
- Practicing yoga asana with full attention

- Practicing activities daily with full attention

Step 4 Concentration

At first you might feel put off at the thought of having so many exercises to practice, and be concerned that the exercises will be too time consuming in your already busy schedule. Be assured that (as you will see in the Appendix F) body awareness, breath awareness attention focus, and concentration and relaxation will be a part of your regular warm-up and cool-down routine. You'll notice that during a few minutes of your regular warm-up you will achieve several tasks at once: practicing relaxation, concentration, attention focus, stretching, physical and mental warm-up, and body and breath awareness. One of the remarkable advantages of yoga is several training tasks can be achieved simultaneously because of the synthesis of mind and body.

There is an interrelationship among the four basic steps (exercises). Body awareness facilitates breath awareness, and conversely, breath awareness facilitates body awareness. Similarly, body and breath awareness facilitate attention focus, and attention focus facilitates breath

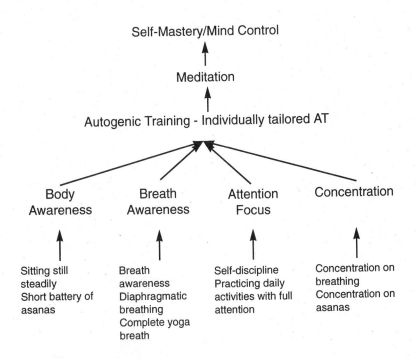

Self-Mastery/Mind Control

↑

Meditation

↑

Autogenic Training - Individually tailored AT

Body Awareness | Breath Awareness | Attention Focus | Concentration

Sitting still steadily
Short battery of asanas

Breath awareness
Diaphragmatic breathing
Complete yoga breath

Self-discipline
Practicing daily activities with full attention

Concentration on breathing
Concentration on asanas

Table 5: Yoga for Self-Mastery

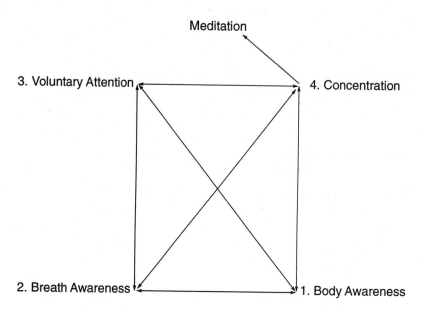

Table 6: Interaction of Basic Steps

and body awareness and lead to the development of concentration. Practicing each of the steps facilitates improvement of the others (Table 6).

After practicing and mastering the four basic steps (exercises), you should start to practice meditation and autogenic training (Table 5). The described techniques, meditation and autogenic training, have the same goal: to extend your potential, to learn autonomic control through passive concentration, to restore and maintain your physical and mental balance, and to alter your inner responses—mind-body synthesis.

Make your program personal, choose exercises you enjoy the most, and you are much more likely to practice diligently. One of the reasons that most athletes chose yoga techniques among the many offered is that practicing yoga produces pleasant feelings. Yoga exercises always rejuvenate and re-energize the body. Keep practicing and you will improve your sports performance and the quality of your life.

Read Appendix F to see how my students incorporated yoga into their daily regimen.

You will find that learning and practicing yoga is easy, feels good and because it affects both mind and body you will simultaneously achieve several training tasks, which is significant in terms of optimum use of training time. You will learn that even with just ten minutes of your daily training practice, you can achieve an integrated mind-body effect.

What is more challenging is systematic, daily practice, commitment to your goals and to yourself—not only your sports achievement goals but also commitment to your physical, mental, and spiritual growth and overall well being. Yoga and the offered program in this book will help you to achieve these goals easier and more effectively.

If your main goal is not achieving top sport results but overall physical, mental, and spiritual growth and well being, then I would suggest you use more time for the practice of yoga asanas and breathing exercises. A program might include 1-2 hours daily of yoga including practicing meditation.

Combining practice of yoga asanas with some type of aerobic, "western," exercises like running, swimming, walking, jogging, biking, etc. is very useful, but it is possible to use some yoga asanas for aerobic workout also.

—— PART 1 ——

YOGA AND SPORT
TRAINING

1

WHAT IS YOGA?

Yoga is the oldest known science of self-development. It is mental, physical and spiritual control. Developed thousands of years ago in India, yoga literally means joining—the joining of the individual self with the universal self. This joining is achieved through the practice and mastering of specific physical postures, called asanas, breathing exercises called pranayama, and meditation—what is known as the path of Raja Yoga, and its subdivision, Hatha Yoga.

There are numerous stories about the remarkable abilities of yogis, those adept in the disciplines of yoga. British doctors more than 200 years ago began studying certain Indians who could do some very unusual and interesting things. These people, called yogis, apparently had phenomenal powers of self-regulation of both mind and body.

In a famous series of scientific experiments at the Menninger Clinic in Topeka, Kansas in 1970, Swami Rama, a spiritual leader from the Himalayas, demonstrated remarkable control over involuntary bodily functions until then considered to be beyond conscious control. Elmer E. and Alyce M. Green, and E. Dale Walters reported that Swami Rama caused two areas about two inches apart on the palm of his right hand to gradually change temperature in opposite directions (at a rate of about four degrees Fahrenheit per minute) until they showed a temperature difference of about ten degrees Fahrenheit. One side of his palm was flushed red with warmth and the other was ashen gray with cold.

In another experiment, Swami Rama raised his heartbeat at will from 70 beats per minute to 300 beats per minute. His heartbeat became a flutter that no longer pumped blood in the normal rhythmic fashion. He also was able to stop his heart for at least 17 seconds. Swami Rama also demonstrated his ability to produce theta waves, when brain waves reach a low 4-7 cycles per second such as during deep meditation or trance. In one five minute period of the test, he produced theta waves 75 percent of the time. He also consciously produced delta waves, when brain waves slow to a mere 0.5 to 3 cycles per second usually during the deepest sleep. (Normal, conscious brain activity is registers between 14 and 28 cycles per second, known as beta waves.) during 25 minutes. After rousing himself he was able to repeat verbatim, all the statements of the experimenters given every five minutes while he was in the delta state. It was believed that in order to produce delta waves one would have to be sound asleep.

As the researchers pointed out in *Biofeedback for Mind/Body Self Regulation, Healing and Creativity* (Plenun Press, 1979): "The importance of Swami Rama's demonstrations did not lie in the performances themselves, but in their implications." Athletes do not intend to practice stopping their heart or to do similar things as Swami Rama, but the fact that it can be done is of major scientific importance. If all athletes became aware that the body responds to self-generated psychological inputs, that heart rate, blood flow, and other body processes can be influenced at will, it would be clear that each athlete could influence his or her own mental and physical preparation. Athletes can realize easier that the pressure, importance of the competition, conditions, etc. is not the problem, but rather, their reaction to it, and this reaction can be to a significant extent self chosen.

It should be stressed that the yogi draws the power for achieving this perfect physical and mental inner harmony, and harmony with the surrounding world, from within.

Profound study of yoga indicates that in all aspects of yoga absolute equilibrium and conscious control of emotions are the emphasized factors. When searching for the principle—the essence—of yoga, we can conclude that its basic principle is to achieve an increased state of concentration and awareness.

The question is: How does the yogi achieve this control? For the athlete, it is important to understand what can be utilized from this ancient self-development science in order to improve the sport performance and training and to achieve physical and mental control.

Studies of yogis who demonstrated unusual control over mind and body, and studies of the mechanisms of involuntary autonomic control indicate that body control is achieved through passive concentration and not through active striving, and the important part of the control is the process and the attention to it—not the outcome nor the goal. These dimensions operate in all physical, emotional, and mental activity.

Yoga helps us learn autonomic control via passive concentration.

In the following pages, I will discuss the most commonly known Hatha Yoga and Raja Yoga exercises. Then, based on experiences in working with many athletes in different sports and of varying performance levels, I will suggest how to improve your sport performance and your well being through yoga.

This book is intended to help you utilize yoga in your sport preparation as well as in your everyday life.

2 ▬▬

HATHA AND RAJA YOGA: TWO PATHS OF TRAINING

The two most popular yoga systems are Hatha Yoga (physical practice) and Raja Yoga (mental exercise). Practice of these yoga forms in the western world are used mostly to develop a healthy and flexible body, improve general health, and to gain self control and inner peace.

Hatha Yoga is composed of exercises for the body. It consists of asanas (body postures), pranayama (breathing exercises), relaxation, and cleansing techniques. There are many styles of Hatha Yoga, but all employ the same basic postures, or asanas, and breathing exercises.

RAJA YOGA

Raja Yoga is a practical system like Hatha Yoga. The objective, however, is to observe, recognize, and control the activity of the nervous system. Raja Yoga is an old technique with many branches.

The *Patanjai's Yoga Sutras* (the first written synthesis of yoga from the second century, B.C.) describes the system of yoga in eight stages:

1. *Yama:* moral, ethical and health guidelines
2. *Niyama:* observances that encourage positive qualities such as purity and contentment
3. *Asanas:* physical postures, exercises to facilitate concentration
4. *Pranayama:* breathing exercises, control of breath

15

5. *Pratyahara*: control of senses, sense withdrawal. The mind is withdrawn from the outside world, from the object of the sense. A final preparation for meditation, the mentioned stages are dealing with the body and the senses. They are basic external preparation—Bahiranga. (Hatha Yoga)

6. *Dharana:* concentration on one object, idea

7. *Dhyana:* meditation, steady concentration on one object, idea

8. *Samadhi:* a state of super-consciousness. The individual self is united with the universal self (The last three stages are higher, internal preparation – Antaranga belonging to Raja Yoga)

Reaching Samadhi is the ultimate goal in yoga. It is in this state that the desired experience of peace and happiness can be attained.

Raja yoga techniques will help you learn autonomic control via passive attention in a more profound way.

During meditation, autogenic training, passive attention, is optimized. In meditation, one learns a focused passive attention without effort, without anticipation. Meditative practices do not focus upon outcome. It is the inspection of the process that is most important.

Raja Yoga techniques will be discussed in other chapters: concentration, meditation, and autogenic training.

HATHA YOGA

Asanas are mostly static body postures that should be executed slowly and without force. Learning and practicing asanas is done step by step and on a regular basis. The postures help you learn autonomic control through passive attention. As Pepper pointed out *Mind/Body Integration* (Plenum Press 1979), "In the asana, the stretch captures our passive attention. Asanas are body attention-getters to bring passive attention to a specific area."

With the asanas, it is possible to work body muscles and keep them in good condition. They can be used deliberately for developing a definite muscle group. The effects can be directed, or localized, in a specific area (muscle group or organ).

The influence of asanas on organ function is rather complicated. For example, in reverse postures the force of gravity is used to attain better circulation and restore proper organ alignment. Function and activity of organs are influenced by asanas in the following ways:

- Increasing pressure inside the body cavities
- Changing cardiovascular pressure and thereby promoting circulation
- Promoting peristalsis which stimulates digestion
- Producing pressure in specific blood vessels in order to regulate circulation
- Stimulating or inhibiting activity of the endocrine glands
- Physically stimulating specific autonomic nerve centers in order to "tune up" the autonomic nervous system, etc.

Asanas are effective for developing correct body posture and for increasing flexibility in joints and the spinal column. They increase strength, endurance, the ability to relax completely, and promote concentration. The asanas fine-tune the nervous and endocrine systems. They stimulate and massage the digestive tract, cardiovascular system, pulmonary organs, and organs of secretion. Asanas directly influence the internal organs, especially the endocrine glands, and by this, influence the metabolism of the organism and overall regeneration.

The most important characteristic of asanas is their static nature. If the postures were dynamic, it would not be possible to achieve the level of concentration and controlled breathing as is possible in the static position.

One of the basic principles of Hatha Yoga is that there is a close relationship/connection between the posture which develops activation by movement (physical activation) and the process of psychical activation. Psychical activation means concentration, conscious participation in the process and the effects of posture in each phase, including the phase of relaxation.

In yoga exercises, the principle of ideomotor reaction is important. Ideomotor reaction is based on the fact that an idea or image can indirectly influence the function of organs, glands, etc. This phenomenon is reinforced by the pull, rotation, and pressure of asanas on the tracks and plexuses of the body.

Another characteristic of yoga exercises in general is slow, fluid, harmonious, and controlled movement, and the coordination of movement with breath, concentration, and body awareness.

The main goal of Hatha Yoga is to facilitate concentration and meditation; that is, preparation for achieving the final stage of yoga—Samadhi.

Normal movements are usually executed mechanically. Often, you see athletes stretching and talking to teammates simultaneously. There is a lack of movement control and introspective feedback. Yoga exercise/stretching is different. It requires concentration, introspection, experiencing and feeling the muscles: the proprioreceptive sensations.

In a posture, the muscles are slowly and gradually stretched into the final position. Here, the subject relaxes while maintaining the position, passively concentrating on the posture's focus point. The subject then returns slowly to the starting position and during relaxation observes and experiences the executed posture. Each yoga posture has its focus point. It can be:

- A muscle, ligament, joint (physiological, effect)
- A vital neuro-vegetative center (chakra) in the body (humoral effect on the organism as a whole)
- The process of relaxation, activation, de-activation (psychological effect)
- Some ideas, images associated with the given asana (spiritual aspect of the asana, spiritual effect)

Each posture has four phases:

1. Controlled, fluent, and slow movement while achieving the final position, and moving back to the starting position (Dynamic phase). The dynamic, or physical part, of the posture (technique) enables correct understanding and memory of the posture.

2. Coordination of movements with breathing (control of breathing). Conscious, controlled breathing promotes unified and harmonious activity in all organs.

3. Passive concentration on the focus point of the posture. Relaxed and motionless (Static phase).

4. Observation and concentration on perceptions and sensations of one's own organism. This enables a high development of self-knowledge as a means of self-control, which also increases the effect of the posture.

This means that one must concentrate during the dynamic phase on:

- Fluid, harmonious, slow, and controlled movements (executing the posture, correct technique).

- Relaxation (relaxation is applied before, during and after the posture). It has specific therapeutic effects on the body and mind. It enables fluid coordination of postures which increases the therapeutic effect.

- Controlled breathing.

and during the static phase on the:

- Focus point of the posture (relaxed motionless).

In each yoga posture, these phases manifest themselves simultaneously and in synchrony. They are mutually related and interdependent.

Achieving the perfect position does not mean achieving "total stretch" or an "acrobatic" position, but mainly that all four parts are in harmony. Therefore, it is necessary to focus first on the dynamic phase (to master the posture, or the controlled movement). Later, the attention should be focused on the breathing and relaxation, then on concentrating on the focus point, and finally on introspection. Then the synchronization of all four phases should be emphasized.

GUIDELINES FOR PRACTICING YOGA ASANAS

I mentioned earlier that learned movements are executed mechanically. Athletes are talking to each other while stretching or jogging. Yoga practice is different.

When starting a posture, be aware of your body. Allow all your muscles to relax. Feel the sensations associated with the contact of part of your body with the floor. Close your eyes and visualize the posture you will assume (mental "tuning"). Assume the posture slowly, smoothly, with full awareness, and concentration moment-to-moment. If your mind wanders, bring it gently back.

Self-suggestive autogenic verbal phrases and mental imagery are also used to affect the body. With these, you will increase the biological effect of the asana on the function of your muscles and organs of the body. For example, repeating in your mind slowly, in a monotone, the autogenic verbal phrase: *Back muscles and/or hamstring muscles stretch.* During the forward bend posture the stretch will be enhanced. After regular practice and repetition of such autosuggestive verbal phrases, the expected reactions will develop in your muscles and body. For example if you repeat in your mind slowly *"My arms are relaxed"* after a while (regular practice) these muscles become actually relaxed.

HOW TO USE AUTOGENIC VERBAL PHRASES

- Repeat the phrases in your mind slowly in a monotone way. After each phrase, pause, then repeat the phrase several more times.

- Concentration on the focal point of the asana, and repetition of the autogenic verbal phrases must be in total harmony.

- The autogenic verbal phrases should enhance the effect of the given asana, increase the asana's biological effect on the given body part or organ on which the concentration is focused.

- Each yoga asana should be executed with total concentration, and with using autogenic verbal phrases.

Do not strive or force your body when attempting a posture. Accept your flexibility, balance, strength, etc. as it is now. When stretching and balancing, listen to your body. Be aware of your sensations. Do not push too far. Do not be achievement oriented or compete for how "far" you can stretch, or how long you can maintain the static phase, etc. Observe, learn your limit. Be aware of the feelings that the posture develops in various parts of your body.

When you get into the final position, maintain it motionless. Maintain each posture long enough to attune, to relax, into the posture. Be aware of your breathing from moment to moment. Feel your belly moving in and out.

A general rule of breathing is that you exhale when you contract your belly and the front side of your body and inhale when you contract your back. For example, if you bend your trunk forward you exhale, when you lean your trunk back you inhale. When maintaining the posture, breathe regularly, feeling your belly moving.

Listen to your body and to your intuition as to how far you should stretch, or how long you should stretch, or how long you should maintain the position. Know your limit, have a non-striving attitude.

As an example, I will guide you through the execution of the forward bend posture (Padhastasana).

FORWARD BEND

MODIFIED PADHASTASANA

Stand in a relaxed position, feet together, trunk straight and arms at your side.

Allow all your muscles to relax. Close your eyes. Be aware of your body. Feel the sensations associated with the contact of your feet with the floor.

Visualize the posture you are going to practice. This is a form of mental tuning.

Inhale, then exhale while you slowly bend forward. Curl down starting at your head and moving through the rest of your spine. Do the movement slowly and in a relaxed manner. From the start to the final position, the movement should be slow, fluid, continuous, and mindful. Bring your hands to the point on your legs or feet that you can reach without strain.

Do not force the stretch. Without effort, let your head and spine lean forward slowly. Just allow your body to bend and the muscles to stretch. Keep your arms, shoulders, neck, and head relaxed and loose. Keep your legs straight, but do not lock your knees.

Grasp your ankles or your legs without effort, and lower your head toward your knees.

Do not strive or force the stretch. Accept your flexibility as it is now. Listen to your body, learn your limit.

Practice with full awareness and concentration, moment to moment.

Be aware of the sensations and feelings the posture develops in different parts of your body, especially in the area of your back and legs.

When you bend forward as far as is comfortable, hold the position motionlessly to attune to the posture. This is referred to as the static position. Breathe slowly and regularly, focusing and feeling the movement of your belly.

Now concentrate on the focal point of this posture, which can be any of the following depending on your goal:

- The hamstring muscle and/or the muscles of the back (physiological aspect of the yoga posture). Repeat in your mind the autogenic verbal phrases: *"My hamstring muscle is stretching," "My back muscles are stretching."*

- The first chakra, called the muladhara chakra, located at the base of the spine. You should direct your attention to the base of the spine, or visualize the symbol of the muladhara chakra: a triangle within a square (humoral aspect of yoga posture). Repeat the autogenic verbal phrase: *"My energy is accumulating."*

- The psychological aspect of the yoga posture, which means concentrating (attuning) on the process of relaxation or deactivation. Repeat in your mind the autogenic verbal phrases: *"My muscles are relaxing," "I am totally relaxed."*

- The spiritual aspect of the yoga posture. Each yoga posture can be associated with some symbol, image, or idea. You can, for example, concentrate on the idea of humility.

After choosing your focal point, just relax into the posture. Attune to your body and mindfully be aware of your feelings and sensations.

Now inhale and return to the starting standing position. Stand up slowly, vertebra by vertebra. Be aware of and feel the changes in your position and in in your spine as you slowly straighten to an erect position. Be aware of the sensations in your body and muscles. Relax. Executing a yoga posture is like meditation. It is more mental than physical.

Relaxation is an important aspect in practicing yoga postures. Relax before, during, and after execution of the posture. Be aware of the nature and characteristics of yoga postures. Learn and practice the described "forward bend" posture. You will use it later. When and which yoga asana to use will be discussed later.

PRANAYAMA

Breathing is connected with bodily functions in a special way. This is one of the facts which makes it possible for yogis to control autonomic functions of the body. By exercising the will and regularly practicing breathing exercises, called pranayama, yogis are able to control organ activities normally controlled by the autonomic nervous system.

The breathing process has special connection with important bodily functions. Therefore, the easiest way to influence these functions is through the control of breathing.

The final goal of most of the yoga breathing exercises is to regulate the mental state by favorably influencing the nervous system. Yoga breathing techniques facilitate concentration and meditation. Through yoga breathing you will gain conscious control over the unconscious activities of the autonomic nervous system.

There is a very tight connection between breathing and emotions. It is likely that you have observed this fact yourself, and it was known even in ancient times. "When the Breath is Still, so is the Mind." This basic yoga concept tell us that, with breathing, we can help to either calm or excite the entire nervous system. When your breath becomes irregular and unsteady, your mental state also becomes unsteady. However, when the breath is steady, so is the mind.

The way that you breathe directly affects your mental and physical state. If you breathe deeply and count silently as you slowly exhale, you can feel yourself relaxing. Try now to breathe irregularly and quickly, and you will feel some anxiety. A surprise or some type of shocking news creates jerks in your breathing, increasing the feelings of anxiety or tension.

"Breathing is the string that controls the kite." According to yoga principles, life is breath. The kite represents the mind, and the breath symbolizes the string. As the breath moves, so moves the mind, just as the string moves with the kite. If breathing is long, slow, and smooth, the mind becomes peaceful.

Through concentration and breathing exercises, yogis are able to control bodily functions that we normally think are out of our control. The yoga system of breathing includes the whole respiratory system. It is slower than ordinary breathing because the lungs are filled completely during each breath. Yoga breathing involves all three methods of breathing: lower (abdominal) breathing, middle (intercostal) breathing, and high (clavicular) breathing.

Each phase of yoga breathing is important and has a specific effect on the mental state. The four phases of yoga breathing are:

1. Inhalation

2. Retaining the breath

3. Exhalation

4. Retaining the breath after exhalation

As mentioned, each phase of yoga breathing influences the mental state in a different way. The exhalation itself has a calming (parasympathetic) effect. Inhalation, followed by extended slow exhalation, brings about a sense of calm and decreases your level of mental excitement.

The response of a specific nerve (the vagus nerve) is actually strengthened when you prolong the exhalation of your breath. The various fibers of the vagus nerve are connected to your lungs and other breathing apparatus. So, when you breathe a slow extended exhalation, the parasympathetic nervous system for calming the body is activated, and your mental state is calmed as well. If the process is reversed and you emphasize the inhalation, then there is a mobilization effect on the body.

Breathing can also be utilized for concentration. You've probably noticed that when you intensely focus your attention on something, you have a tendency to hold your breath. If you retain your breath, your mind tends to become focused ("one-point"). If your breath is irregular, your mind becomes scattered.

Smooth, rhythmic, harmonious breathing—with focused attention—can help you to develop a much higher level of concentration. One of the explanations for this effect might be that the center for breathing is located in the part of the brain where all the important centers for life are located. The centers that control muscle tone, heart movement, blood circulation, and concentration are all located in the reticular formation of the brain. Variations in breathing can affect these other centers, and also affect your concentration and the functions of the nervous system.

LEARNING YOGIC BREATHING

The following exercises are presented in the order in which you should master them. First, you should learn abdominal breathing. Next, you should learn the technique of breath awareness (deep, natural, smooth, rhythmic diaphragmatic breathing). Then, learn alternate nostril breathing. The above mentioned breathing exercises can be learned from the description. They do not require an instructor, and are sufficient for achieving your goals. Be aware that more advanced pranayama exercises can be harmful if not used properly. If you wish to practice more advanced techniques, you should see a qualified instructor. These exercises cannot be learned from a book.

ABDOMINAL BREATHING

Sit comfortably with head, neck, and trunk erect and in a straight line. Exhale slowly and smoothly and contract your abdominal muscles. As you exhale, the stomach moves inward. Now relax your abdomen and slowly and smoothly inhale. As you inhale, the stomach moves outward, pushing your abdominal muscles forward slightly arching your lower back. Now exhale again. By contracting your abdominal muscles, the stomach moves inward and flattens your back. Repeat this several times. Breathe through your nose, smoothly and steadily.

Put your hands on your stomach and feel your stomach moving in and out as you are breathing. This will help you learn the proper technique. It is very important to practice abdominal breathing to learn how to use the diaphragm and breathe smoothly and deeply. It will also help you to learn how to relax the abdominal muscles when they become tense due to stress. Abdominal breathing is the most important part of the complete yoga breath that you are going to learn. Practice diaphragmatic breathing 5-10 minutes two times daily to master it.*

BREATH AWARENESS

Sitting in a still and steady position with the head, neck, and trunk erect, relax all your muscles. Now focus your attention to your breathing. Visualize and mentally follow the flow of the breath. It should be natural, deep, smooth, rhythmic, and diaphragmatic without noise, pauses, and holding the breath.

Just follow mentally the flow of your smooth breathing. The length of inhalation should be equal with the length of exhalation. Do not hold your breath or have pauses between inhalation and exhalation. Do not force your breathing; make your breathing silent, noiseless.

Become aware of your belly moving in and out, and the air entering and leaving the nostrils.

Practice breath awareness two times daily for 10-15 minutes. You can practice while sitting or while walking. After a month of practicing breath awareness, you can prolong the exhalation twice the length of your inhalation. For example, if you inhale to a count of six, exhale to a count of twelve, etc.

COMPLETE YOGA BREATH

As mentioned earlier, yoga recognizes three types of breathing: low (abdominal), middle (inter-costal), and high (clavicular). From a physiological point of view, complete breathing is the most effective because it combines the effects of all three kinds of breathing.

---

* Practice abdominal breathing while reclining flat on the floor. Place a heavy book on your stomach to strengthen your diaphragm muscles. A similar effect can be achieved by lying on your stomach with the forehead resting on your forearm. In this case the floor will provide resistance.

To start complete yoga breathing, assume a comfortable sitting position with the head, neck, and trunk erect and in a straight line. All breathing is done through the nose. Slowly execute a deep exhalation as described in abdominal breathing. Now, distend your abdomen pushing forward with you abdominal muscles, and slowly, quietly, in hale. Air is pouring almost without effort into the lower part of the lungs. Slightly arch your lower back. (This is low abdominal or diaphragmatic breathing, which you have already learned.) Inhaling slowly, smoothly, and quietly, bring your extended abdomen or stomach in until it feels taut. At the same time, spread your rips and your entire rib cage forward and out to the side. (This is middle, or inter-costal, breathing.)

Continue your slow inhalation. While you do, keep your chest extended and fill the upper part of your lungs. (This is high, or clavicular, breathing.) Feel the breath hitting the back of your throat and hear the steam-like sound as you inhale and exhale. Now, exhale slowly, smoothly and quietly. Lower your shoulders, contract the chest and move your stomach inward. Swami Rama suggests visualizing that you are breathing from the base of the spine to the crown of the head as you inhale, and as you exhale visualize the breath leaving from the crown of your head down through the spine, smoothly and evenly.

Practice the complete yoga breath for a few weeks to master it. To better control the breathing and to achieve greater smoothness, A. Christensen suggests that you wear ear plugs. You will increase the evenness and smoothness of your breath, and your concentration will increase as well.

After learning the complete yoga breath, you can use it anytime, anywhere to calm your mind and to fight stress.

ALTERNATE NOSTRIL BREATHING

Sit in a still and steady position. Relax all your muscles. Calm your body.

Place the tip of your thumb against your right nostril. Fold your index and middle fingers together. Place the tip of your ring finger against your left nostril. Exhale deeply through both nostrils.

Now, close your right nostril, by gently pressing your thumb against it. Leave your left nostril open. Now inhale, taking a smooth, deep, complete yoga breath through your left nostril. Next, gently close your left nostril with your ring finger, remove your thumb from your right nostril and exhale slowly, evenly through your right nostril. Then, inhale through your right nostril. Close your right nostril gently with your index finger. Remove your ring finger and exhale through your left nostril. Then, again inhale through your left nostril. Close your left nostril. Remove your thumb and exhale through your right nostril, etc. Breathing should be smooth and diaphragmatic, even with equal length of inhalation and exhalation. Each time that you return to the original point (that is, inhaling through your left nostril), you have completed one series of alternate nostril breathing.

Practice for about six to eight weeks two times daily with ten series of alternate nostril breathing.

Alternate nostril breathing is used as preparation for meditation, because it calms the mind and produces a state suitable for meditation.

THE RECHARGING AND RELEASING BREATH (THE "DOUBLE R" BREATH)

Take a deep, slow complete yoga breath and visualize that with this breath you are recharging, accumulating your energy, or prana.

Now, slowly exhale. As you do this, visualize that you are releasing the tension in the muscles of your face, neck, shoulders, trunk, thighs, and calves in that order.

Visualize, that with releasing the muscle tension, you simultaneously release the negative emotions and thoughts.

Use the "Double R" breath whenever you feel tension or have lost your focus.

RELAXATION

In yoga, relaxation is employed before, during, and after practicing asanas. The student learns how to relax his or her inner tensions and in fact applies this technique to live a relaxed life.

The yogi starts relaxation exercise in the Savasana, or corpse, posture—laying back, with legs comfortably extended, arms beside the trunk and eyes closed. The yogi then relaxes all muscles and eliminates tension step by step. During this time of relaxation, the yogi temporarily disconnects his or her consciousness with the rest of the world. He or she can gradually distinguish even the smallest amount of tension in muscles and mind. The Yogi experiences an inner self awareness from within the muscles, ligaments, and internal organs. At this point, it is possible to begin controlling the autonomic activities of the central nervous system by concentrating on the spontaneous breathing process without disturbing the rhythm of breathing. Simultaneously, a correlating change can be observed in the heart's activity.

This technique allows us to experience a phenomenon of looseness and calmness. In fact, true yoga practice starts when peace and relaxation of physical being is followed by that of the nervous system as a result of discovering inner self awareness.

Relaxation will be discussed further in the chapter of autogenic training, kinesthetic training, and body control.

3

YOGA FOR SPORTS AND WELLNESS

Physical preparation for maintaining optimum fitness, technical preparation for improving your sports skills, and tactical preparation for developing strategy and tactical skills require a lot of time. Daily mental skills (relaxation techniques, concentration, imagery) to control your mental state must also be practiced. If you take into account the time you need for study or work (or both) and for your, social life, the time aspect is crucial. From these aspects, yoga is a very effective means of training. It affects the mind/body simultaneously and harmoniously.

I observed during many years of working with athletes, both as coach and psychologist, that yoga is the most effective means in accomplishing the daily practice of mental skills. Incorporating one or two asanas into your regular warm-up and/or cool-down routine provides several mental benefits in addition to the usual physical effects. You practice attention-concentration relaxation (a mental skill) while simultaneously stretching and warming-up (or down) your body, increasing flexibility and body awareness. You also mentally tune yourself. Yoga concentration is a "transition" to the concentration required (and so important) for performance or training. Also, just as warm-up and cool-down is part of the athlete's everyday routines, mental skill practice becomes a regular, systematic habit of the athlete. Incorporating yoga in your cool-down routine will also simultaneously speed up the recovery (regeneration) process. (See Yoga Regeneration Exercises in Chapter 4)

The most wonderful thing about practicing yoga is that besides all the mentioned benefits it produces a very pleasant feeling, regenerating, rejuvenating the mind/body. Athletes claim they feel re-energized after practicing yoga.

YOGA'S MANY USES

Athletes can use yoga asanas and pranayama for different purposes (see also Tables 2, 3, 5, and 6 in the Introduction):

- For promoting general health, prevention of bad health as part of a healthy lifestyle.
- For speeding up the process of regeneration after training and competition and for rehabilitation.
- For correcting the muscle dysbalance as a result of a one-sided training load, by overall harmonization of the organism.
- For increasing flexibility and elasticity, for warm-up, and warm-down.
- For increasing strength, especially when concentrating on a definite muscle or muscle groups.
- For developing self-observation, body awareness, self-study, self-discipline.
- For developing attention, concentration.
- For calming the mind and making it joyful.

Athletes can utilize Raja Yoga techniques in their psychological preparation:

- For improving relaxation, attention concentration.
- For learning autonomic control through passive attention.
- For mind/body self-regulation.

4

YOGA AS TRAINING EXERCISES

In this chapter you will learn the benefit of incorporating Hatha Yoga into your training.

In Chapter 6 you will find a number of asanas constructed for different purposes, like: "YRE for Short Term Rest," "Asanas to Prevent Pain and Back Injury," "YRE For Releasing Shoulder Tension," "The Double "R" Breath in Case of High Stress." In Chapter 8 you will learn how to construct a battery of asanas for your own specific needs. You will gain a clear understanding how you can use these supplemental, compensational, and regenerative exercises for your own specific needs in your sport training.

You will learn how to use yoga for improving, practicing mental skills like concentration, relaxation, and imagery—for mind/body control. You will learn the steps for achieving mind control—self-mastery through yoga. You will also find examples of how to incorporate yoga in your daily sport training.

YOGA SUPPLEMENTAL EXERCISES (YSE)

Yoga Supplemental Exercises (YSE) are an important means of preparation in each sport. Supplemental training means practicing sports and activities other than your sport in order to build overall fitness. Such overall fitness usually cannot be achieved with the practice of just a single sport. The reasons for practicing supplemental training (exercises and activities) include the following:

- Some sports develop only a limited range of muscles (for example, fencing alone develops a certain group of muscles more than others).

- Beginning competition at an early age can negatively influence the harmonious development of the young child. Supplemental training is necessary to assure harmonious development, and supplemental exercises are a good habit to develop in a young athlete for they help develop a strong base on which to build specific abilities.

- Increased training load along with a prolonged preparation period and extensive competitive period also puts high pressure on the nervous system. Supplemental training creates a desirable "switch-off" mechanism for the physical and mental stress accumulated from this.

Yoga Supplemental Exercises are an effective means of avoiding monotony and boredom in a training program. It also helps avoid overtraining while providing variety and fun in the routine. YSE, in the form of "active rest," balances the training load. Competition along with everyday stress taxes the nervous system and depletes mental stamina. YSE are an effective means of restoring energy and physical and mental equilibrium. YSE also promote health while assuring harmonious physical and mental development.

Section Two, which contains photos and instructions of each posture, delineates which asanas are used for what type of exercises.

YOGA COMPENSATION EXERCISES (YCE)

As a result of long-term sport training, muscle dysbalance can develop in the athlete's body. The cardiovascular and pulmonary system are usually loaded as a unit, but the different muscle groups are loaded individually. Partial loading occurs when some muscle groups are neglected, not strengthened during training. Only partial loading of the muscles takes place, depending on the given sport. The muscle groups become unbalanced either by overloading certain muscle groups through "one-sided" training, or by weakening some muscle groups through lack of involvement or practice. In fencing, for example, the non-weaponed arm, and the leg and trunk on the non-weaponed side become less developed than the other side. Such "one-sided" loading produces damage, disturbance, and injury to the motoric system. An effort must be made to avoid this dysbalance in order to ensure overall fitness.

The task of YCE is to correct and compensate for the developed muscle dysbalance by regular, systematic practice of compensation exercises. YCE corrects the one-sided effect of training by promoting general harmonious development of the body and by improving the individual physical systems.

Overall, yoga has the effect of compensating and correcting the dysbalance which results from one-sided loading of the muscles. Yoga exercises are the most complex, rational, and complete activity for overcoming the one-sided effects of loading. Learning the different YCE asanas and their effects as well as becoming aware of the insufficiently loaded muscle groups by your sport will enable you to select the appropriate asanas for compensation of the muscle dysbalances.

YOGA REGENERATION EXERCISES (YRE)

Successfully completing long and intensive athletic training for achieving top performance depends largely on the extent to which the athlete can regenerate his/her physical and mental strength after training. Not surprisingly, top sport performance requires hard, intensive training. Without fast and profound muscle regeneration, it is impossible to withstand a daily, rigorous regimen.

After intensive training or competition, it is necessary to immediately start the process of regeneration. Regeneration is a biological process fostered by athletes for regaining strength and prevention of injuries. It is an inseparable part of sport preparation. Yoga Regeneration Exercises (YRE) are useful here.

With a truly committed implementation of regeneration methods, it is possible to decrease muscle fatigue by 30 percent and to increase the intensity of training by 20 percent, according to Eastern European experts J. Liska, M.D. and L Zbojan, M.D. in their study *Specificke Prostriedky*

Regeneracie (Specific Means of Regeneration) Metodicke Listy Suv CSTV, Bratislava, 1987.

Regeneration has many benefits for athletes. Among the most important are:

- Restoration of strength after loading
- Fast elimination of the symptoms of fatigue especially in the muscles. (Restoring the "millieo interior" of the body, the equilibrium function of the higher nervous system)
- Prevention of injury to permanently loaded muscle groups

These benefits make possible a significant increase in the effectiveness of the entire training process. They facilitate the development of correct sports skills, movement habits, and protect the body of the athlete, thereby increasing the overall effectiveness of an economical training regimen.

For all these reasons and benefits, it becomes clear why top athletes pay special attention to the regeneration process. YRE positively influences this process. Psychologically, yoga exercises generally optimize passive attention, which leads to greater autonomic control. Yoga exercises "gather" attention, as in meditation, enabling the regeneration of the entire body by developing a favorable mental state (parasympathetic dominance).

Physically, YRE are the most important means of active muscle regeneration. This system of selected or modified yoga exercises relaxes the loaded, stiff, and shortened muscles that are the product of hard training or competition. These exercises speed up the regeneration of the frequently loaded muscle groups.

There are three basic types of muscle relaxation, all of which are included in YRE:

- Stretching—relaxation of the shortened and painful muscles by stretching.
- Post-isometric relaxation (PIR) (semi-active method)—executed usually with the assistance of a therapist or teammate. PIR is a relaxation which develops after isometric tension of

muscles for a duration of 10-30 seconds against a low resistance. This active stretching of muscles induces inhibition of motorneurons and the related muscles which significantly facilitates the release of muscles in the phase of relaxation (it seems that the body induces a defensive inhibition against over-loading. For example, such inhibition of motorneurons force the wrestler to terminate a "bridge" position).

- Anti-gravitational relaxation (AGR)—an active method of auto-relaxation. It is a modification of the above mentioned PIR, which substitutes the resistance provided by the therapist or teammate during the isometric tension with the weight of the athlete's own limbs, or trunk, according to Liska and Zbojan. It also uses the natural resistances against which the muscles are isometrically contracted, held for 15-20 seconds, and released (such as elevated limbs, trunk, etc.). This is a simple method the athlete can do without aids. The goal is to develop muscle relaxation following the phase of muscle contraction.

YRE are based on the principle that muscles will release and relax after stretching for a specific time period in a tense and isometric position against specific resistance. This results in inhibition of motorneurons. This "post-isometric relaxation" differs from common stretching exercises which passively stretch the shortened muscles without deliberate (conscious) focus on influencing motorneurons.

YRE significantly influences the vital neuro-vegetative plexuses (chakras) and the endocrine glands. By doing this, the metabolism and overall regeneration of the athlete is positively enhanced.

Method of Practice

YRE

Practice YRE immediately after the training process or competition, in the gym or on the sport field. This immediate phase of regeneration should last 5-15 minutes.

Practice the YRE with passive concentration. Maintain the final static position motionless for 4-10 deep breaths (10-20 seconds). (see Chapter 6)

YSE

Select a battery of YSE and practice them at home, or outdoors. (see Chapter 6)

YCE

Similarly as YSE. (see Chapter 6)

In Section Two, I present a number of YSE, YCE, and YRE. These exercises have been successfully used by many top as well as junior level athletes.

You should select a battery of asanas according to your sport and your needs. Examples are given of how some world-class athletes selected their batteries.

PART II
ASANAS

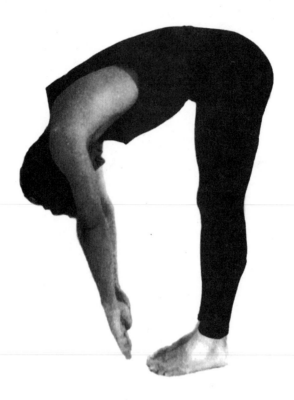

THE MODIFIED STANDING FORWARD BEND

5 ▰

YOGA ASANAS:
HOW TO ACHIEVE THE POSTURES

The following are asanas most frequently incorporated into the workout programs used by athletes I have trained. Each description of each posture is accompanied by a photo or photos. The instructions include the function of the asana—YRE, YSE or YCE.

THE MODIFIED STANDING FORWARD BEND
(MODIFIED PADA HASTHASANA)

Stand in a relaxed posture with feet slightly apart. The trunk is straight, arms at sides. Bend forward slowly without bending the legs at the knees. Do not lock the knees. Push your shoulders slightly forward. Bring hands toward the floor without strain. Use the force of gravity for isometric contraction of the hamstring and back muscles. Maintain this position for several deep breaths. Then, relax and curl up into a standing position. The knee flexor muscles are affected here—isometrically contracted (YRE, YCE).

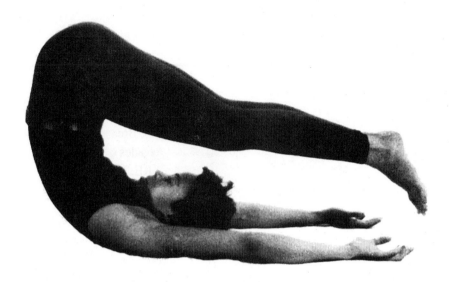

THE HALF PLOUGH

THE HALF PLOUGH
(MODIFIED HALASANA)

Lie on your back, arms at your sides. Raise your legs slowly to a vertical position. Now raise your waist and hips from the floor and bring your legs back over your head until they are about 5-10 inches above the floor. Bring your arms above your head. This increases the effect of gravity. Maintain this position for several deep breaths while you feel the increasing effects of gravity. Then relax. You may continue from this position to the next position: the half shoulderstand. The muscles of the back and rear thighs are affected here – isometrically contracted. (YRE, YCE)

THE HALF SHOULDERSTAND
(MODIFIED SARVANGASANA)

Lie on your back, arms at your sides. Raise your legs slowly to a vertical position. Now raise your waist and hips from the floor supporting the hips with your hands. Your legs are approximately 60 degrees to the floor. The toes line up slightly behind the head. By pressing the hips forward, the force of gravity on the back muscles is increased. Breathe deeply. Maintain this position for several deep breaths. The muscles of the back and the knee flexors are affected—isometric tension. (YRE, YCE, YSE)

You may continue from this position to sitting forward bend.

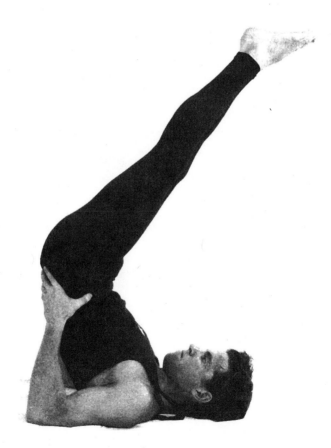

THE HALF SHOULDERSTAND

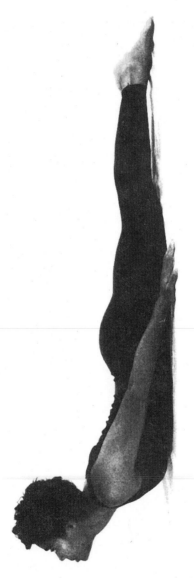

THE MODIFIED COBRA

THE MODIFIED COBRA
(MODIFIED BHUJANGASANA)

Lie on your abdomen. Rest your forehead on the floor, with arms at your side. Inhale. Slowly tilt the head backward—maintain this position for 3-4 deep breaths, then raise your shoulders, trunk and back from the floor. Maintain this position for several deep breaths. Breathe regularly and contract your abdominal muscles while maintaining the final position. Do not use your arms to help. Release the position, lie flat, and relax. (Gradual isometric tension of the upper, middle and lower part of back muscles. Here again the elevated trunk is used for isometric tension.)

The upper, middle and lower muscles of the spine are gradually affected—isometrically contracted. (YRE, YCE)

The Locust

(Salabhasana)

Lie on your abdomen; rest your chin on the floor; make two fists and place them under you just even with the pelvic girdle. Inhale. Push down with your fists and raise both legs 5-15 inches above the floor. Maintain this position for several deep breaths. Release the position then lie flat on the abdomen and relax. The muscles of the back and hamstrings are affected – isometrically contracted.

Here the elevated limbs are used for isometric contractions of muscles. (YRE, YCE, YSE).

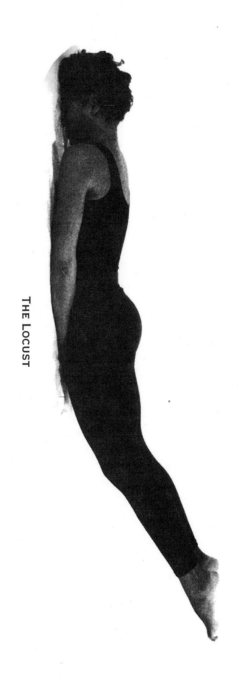

THE LOCUST

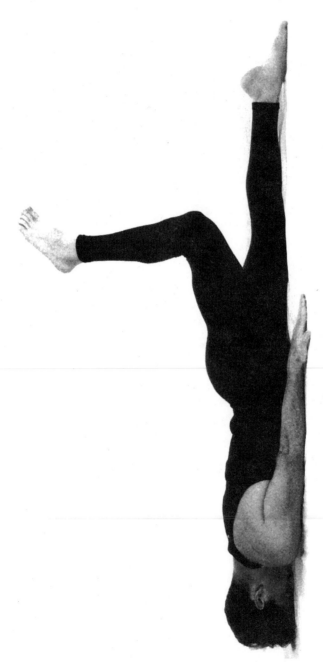

THE MODIFIED HALF LOCUST

THE MODIFIED HALF LOCUST
(MODIFIED SALABHASANA)

This is an easier variation on the previous exercise. Lie in the same position as for the Locust, with hands palms down beside the body. Inhale. Raise your right leg 5-10 inches above the floor. The right knee should be bent approximately 45 degrees. Maintain this position for several deep breaths, then repeat with the left leg. Relax, lying face down. The back muscles and hamstrings on the chosen side are affected – isometrically contracted. (YRE, YCE)

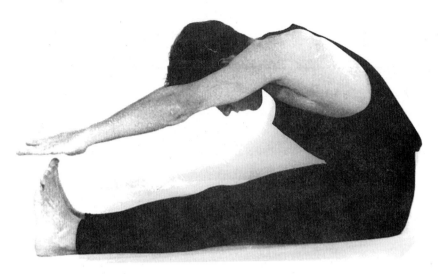

MODIFIED SITTING FORWARD BEND

MODIFIED SITTING FORWARD BEND
(MODIFIED PASCHIMOTHANASANA)

(This posture is often executed immediately after the half shoulderstand. To do this, first slowly lower hips and back to the floor, then also your legs.) Lie on your back. Now gently sit up. Sit with legs straight out before you. Raise your arms slowly, bend, and reach forward with extended arms 5-10 inches above your toes. By doing this, the effect of gravity is increased but mediated by the weight of the trunk and head. Maintain this position for several deep breaths. Then relax in a sitting position.

The muscles of the back and hamstrings are affected—isometrically contracted. The abdominal muscles are also strengthened and the organs in the stomach area receive a gentle massage. This is one of the most effective exercises for relaxing the hamstrings and back muscles (YRE, YCE).

THE TWISTING POSITION
(MODIFIED PARIVARTHANASANA)

Lie on your back. Bend your knees. Place your right heel on your left knee (on the outer side of the knee). Now turn your hips to the right side close to the floor keeping your legs crossed and with your heel on your knee. While you turn, extend your left arm at shoulder level. Now grab your left shoulder with your right hand. Turn your head, especially your chin, to the left. Maintain the position for several breaths at the point you feel the greatest tension in your spine. Then relax lying down on your back. Repeat on the other side. The spine muscles are affected (YRE, YCE).

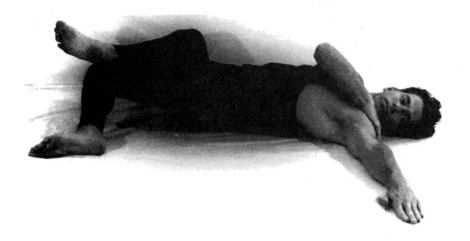

THE TWISTING POSITION

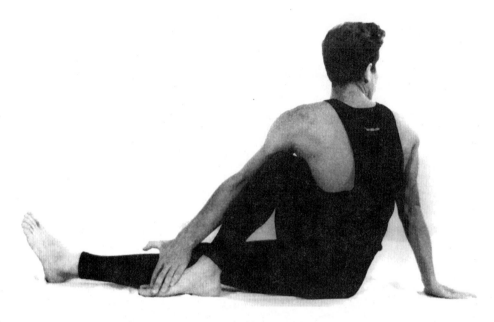

THE TWIST

THE TWIST

(MODIFIED ARDHA MATSYENDRASANA)

Sit with legs straight out in front of you. Bend your right knee and put your right foot over the left knee on the floor. Put your left elbow over your right knee and fix your right knee firmly, tensing the lower part of the spine. Turn your right shoulder to the right. Support yourself with your right arm on the floor behind your back. Breathe deeply, and after each exhalation, increase the degree of twist by moving your right arm further back. Maintain this position for several breaths. The entire spine is affected. Repeat on the opposite side (YRE, YCE).

THE TREE POSTURE
(MODIFIED VRIKSHASANA)

Stand erect. Place the right foot as high on the left inner thigh as possible. Raise your arms above your head. Repeat with the left foot. The effect of the exercise can be increased by bending the trunk forward. Maintain for several deep breaths. The ankle and knees are affected (YRE, YCE).

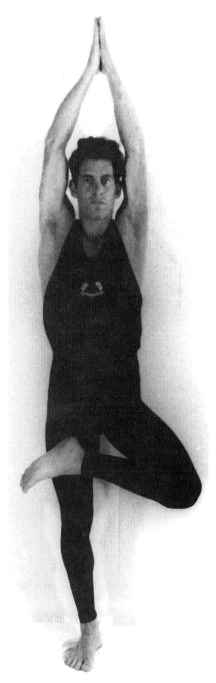

THE TREE

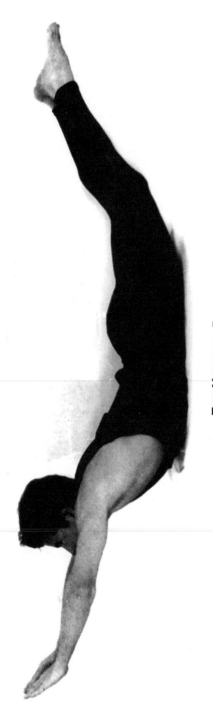

THE MODIFIED BOW

THE MODIFIED BOW

(MODIFIED DHANURASANA)

Lie on your abdomen, face down, arms above your head. Inhale. Raise your head, shoulders, arms, and legs above the floor. Maintain this position for several deep breaths. Relax. The muscles of the back and hamstrings are affected—isometrically contracted. Also, the spine elasticity and tone of the abdominal organs is enhanced. The elevated limbs, head, and trunk are used for isometric contractions (YRE, YCE).

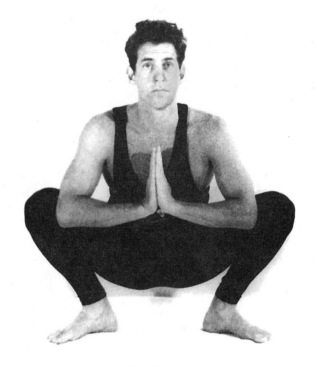

THE FROG

THE FROG

Stand relaxed but erect, feet 15-20 inches apart, with toes pointed outward. Slowly go into a squatting position. Raise your arms and bend your elbows. Bring your palms together against your chest. Press your elbows outward against your knees as far as possible. Maintain for several breaths, then relax and rise to a standing position. The ankle and knee joints are affected (YRE, YCE).

THE EAGLE POSTURE
(GARUDASANA)

Stand erect with feet together. Bend the right knee. Bring the left leg over the right thigh above the right knee and rest the back of the left thigh on the front of the right thigh. Bring the left foot behind the right calf so that the left shin touches the back of the right calf. Bend the arms at the elbow and raise them to chest level. Rest the right elbow on the front of the left upper arm near the elbow joint, then move the right hand back to the right and the left hand forward to the left so as to join palms. Now lift your body off the floor as high as possible, reaching upward.

Strong radical stretch occurs in all the body's joints. Maintain for several deep breaths, then relax in a standing position. All the joints of the body are affected. (YRE, YCE)

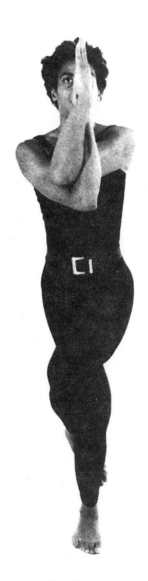

THE EAGLE

THE DANCER'S POSTURE
(MODIFIED NATARAJASANA)

Stand erect. Bend your right knee and raise your right leg so that you can grasp the right foot with your right hand. Wrap your fingers and thumb around your ankles. Raise your left arm straight above your head. Now pull your right leg up and back away from your body, as slowly and as high as you can. Fix your eyes steadily on a spot. This will help you maintain your balance. Relax your abdominal muscles, breathe easily. Feel the stretch (contraction) of the muscles in your thigh. Raise your left arm above the head. Maintain the position for several deep breaths. Relax in a standing position. Now do the same with the left leg. The quadriceps of the thigh, calves, and buttocks are affected. Sense of balance is enhanced. (YRE, YCE)

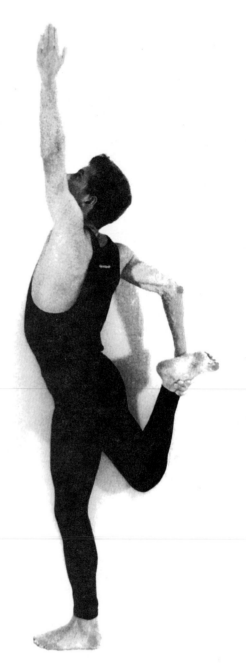

THE DANCER'S POSTURE

THE TRIANGLE
(MODIFIED TRIKONASANA)

Stand erect with feet apart, arms out to me side at shoulder level, and palms facing down. Turn your left foot 90 degrees to the left and the right foot 30 degrees to the left. Bend your trunk to the left slowly and touch the left foot with your left hand as close to the ground as you can. Stretch. Hold it. Maintain for several deep breaths. Slowly return to the standing position. Do not bend the legs or arms when bending down or when getting up. Repeat now on the opposite side. (YRE, YCE)

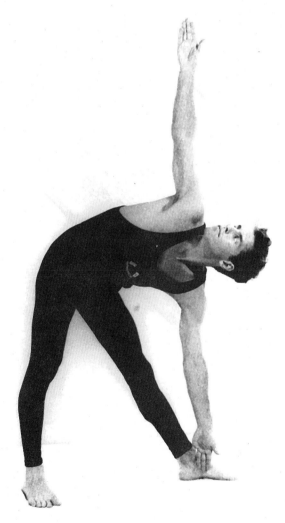

THE TRIANGLE

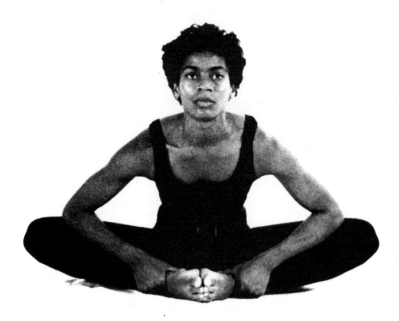

THE GROIN STRETCH

THE GROIN STRETCH

(MODIFIED BHADRASANA)

Sit with legs straight in front of you Bring the soles of the feet together and bring the feet in about one foot away from your body. Sit erect, grasp your ankles with your hands. Inhale. Straighten your spine. Then exhale, lean forward while pressing the knees downward with your elbows. Maintain for several breaths, then repeat. Relax. (YRE, YCE)

THE HALF LOTUS
(MODIFIED PADMASANA)

Sit with your legs straight out in front of you. Place the left foot as high on the right thigh as possible. The right leg is still extended. Press the left knee toward the floor with your left hand. Maintain for several breaths. Then relax in a sitting position with legs bent. Do the same with the opposite leg. The ankles and knees are affected. (YRE, YCE)

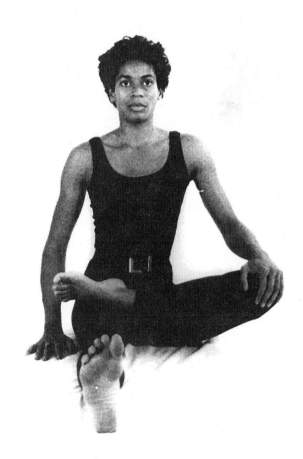

THE HALF LOTUS

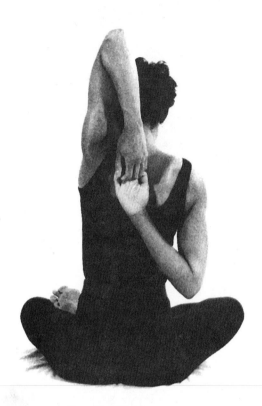

THE SHOULDER STRETCH

THE SHOULDER STRETCH
(MODIFIED GOMUKHASANA)

(STANDING OR SITTING) Raise your right hand and bring it behind your shoulder. Now bend the left hand behind the back from the bottom and join your hands (fingers) together. Now pull up with the top arm and down with the bottom arm gently. Hold for several breaths. Then release the hands and repeat on the other side. Use a towel, t-shirt, or belt to pull arms closer together if you are unable to join hands behind you. The shoulders, hands, arms, and chest are affected. (YRE, YCE)

THE CHEST EXPANSION

Stand erect. Move your arms outward and then straight back behind your back as far as possible. (Step 1) Clasp hands, fingers interlaced, and straighten arms. Gently bend backward from the waist and hold for 3 breaths. Bring clasped arms up over the back and bend deep forward from the waist as you exhale. Lift the arms up and away from your body. (Step 2) Relax the neck. Maintain for several breaths. Relax in a standing position. The chest and shoulders are affected. (YRE, YCE)

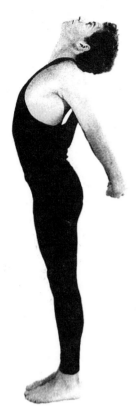

**THE CHEST EXPANSION
STEP 1**

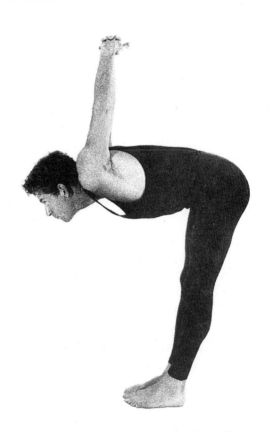

THE CHEST EXPANSION STEP 2

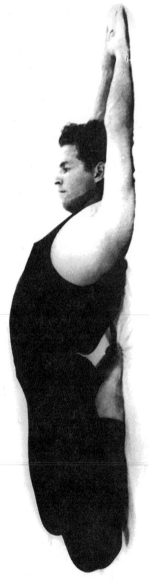

THE RESTING POSTURE

THE RESTING
POSTURE
(MODIFIED VAJRASANA)

Kneel on the floor while sitting on your heels (tops of feet flat on the floor). Keeping your knees on the floor, with the help of the elbows, slowly lean backward so as to be on your back. Lie flat on the floor. Stretch your arms above your head. Relax in this position and maintain it for several breaths. Make sure the back of your head and shoulders rest flat on the floor and your knees are together. The feet, knees, pelvic region and abdominal organs are affected. (YRE, YCE)

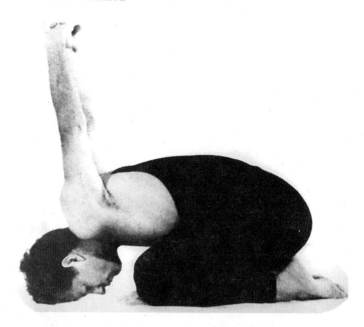

THE MODIFIED CHEST EXPANSION

THE MODIFIED CHEST EXPANSION
(MODIFIED YOGA MUDRA)

Assume a kneeling position and sit on your heels, or a cross-legged position. Bring your arms behind your back, and interlock your fingers. Inhale and bend forward at the waist, at the same time raising your arms straight up behind you, keeping your hands clasped. Exhale and slowly bend forward, keeping your hands clasped. The forehead touches the floor. Hold for several seconds, then come back to the starting position and relax. Repeat 2-3 times.

YOGA SUPPLEMENTAL EXERCISES (YSE)

The following asanas offer an entire body effect. They stimulate the endocrine, nervous, and circulatory systems, and produce an overall positive effect on the nervous system (on mental "Regeneration") as well. (Many of these exercises can be used also as YRE or YCE)

THE SHOULDERSTAND
(SARVANGASANA)

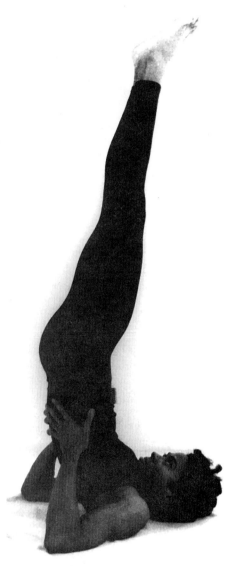

Lie on your back with arms at your sides. Inhale; exhale and raise your legs slowly to a vertical position and then continue to raise your legs and hips, putting your legs directly over your head. Place your palms against the back as close to the shoulders as possible. The elbows are on the floor supporting the trunk. Press your breast bone against your chin. Keep your legs straight, relaxed and perpendicular to the floor. Breathe evenly. Hold for several deep breaths. Exhale and slowly lower your legs and hips to the starting position. Relax.

This posture has a many-sided effect on regeneration. It influences the entire body with a stimulating effect on all organs of the body. Blood supply is increased to all structures of the neck; the thyroid and parathyroid glands are also stimulated.

The focus point is on the thyroid gland.

THE SHOULDERSTAND

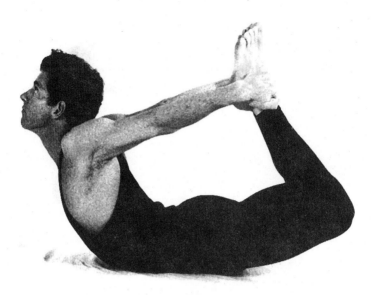

THE BOW

THE BOW

(DHANURASANA)

Lie on your stomach, placing your forehead on the floor with arms at your sides. Bend both legs at the knees. Reach back and grasp both ankles. Inhale; raise your head, shoulders, and chest. Pull on your ankles, lifting the knees as high off the floor as possible. Breathe evenly. Maintain this position for several deep breaths. Exhale. Slowly lower the legs and torso to the starting position. Relax. Repeat 2-3 times.

The bow increases flexibility of the spine, stretches the abdominal muscles, and strengthens the knee joints. The bow also affects the solar plexus, thyroid gland, liver, kidneys, adrenaline gland, pancreas, and the sexual glands.

The focus point is on the solar plexus.

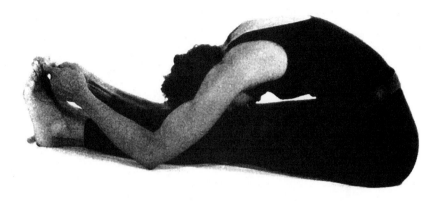

THE SEATED FORWARD BEND

THE SEATED FORWARD BEND
(PASCHIMOTHANASANA)

Sit on the floor with your trunk and head straight, and with your legs straight out before you. Inhale, raise your arms slowly, bend forward and reach forward with extended arms as far as comfortable. Grasp your toes (or ankles or shins if you can't reach your toes). Bring your head to your knees. Breath evenly. Maintain this position for several deep breaths. Then inhale and slowly come back to the starting position.

The muscles of the back and the hamstrings are affected. This is one of the most effective exercises for relaxing the hamstrings and the muscles of the back. The abdominal muscles are also affected. The organs in the abdomen are receiving gentle massage. This stimulates peristaltic movement, as well as kidney, liver, stomach, spleen, and pancreas function. Flexibility of the spine is also increased. The focus point is on the hamstring and back muscles.

THE PLOUGH

(HALASANA)

(This posture can be a continuation of the shoulderstand.) Lie on your back with arms at your sides. Inhale, exhale and slowly raise both legs vertical to the floor, then continue to raise your legs and hips up over your head until your toes touch the floor behind your head. Breathe evenly. Maintain this position for several deep breaths. Then exhale and slowly lower the hips and legs to the starting position.

The plough relaxes the muscles of the back and thighs, stretches the ligaments of the spinal column, stimulates and tones all internal organs, enhances blood circulation, and reduces fatigue. Overall, it is a relaxing, reviving posture.

The focus point is on the spine.

THE PLOUGH

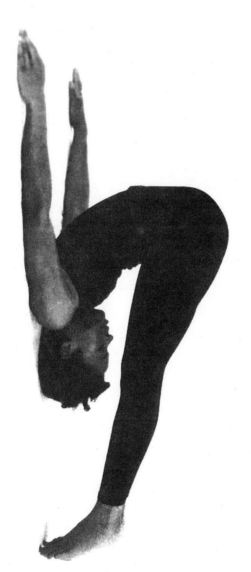

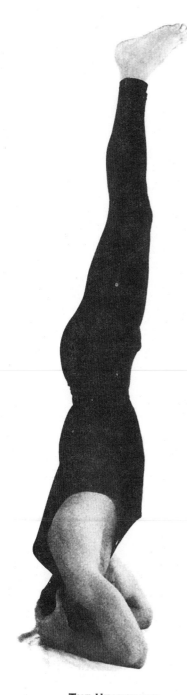

THE HEADSTAND
(SIRSHASANA)

Sit in a kneeling position. Place your arms on the floor in front of you in a triangular position. Interlace your fingers. Raise your hips slightly and place the crown of your head on the floor. Support the upper back of your head with your interlaced fingers. Lift your knees off the floor and walk the feet toward the body until the back is perpendicular to the floor. Raise both legs, bringing your knees toward your chest and your heels toward your buttocks. Slowly raise your legs until they are perpendicular to the floor. Breathe evenly and hold this position for several deep breaths. Then, reversing this sequence, come back to the starting position. The focus point is on the pineal gland.

This asana is considered the king of the asanas in Hatha Yoga. It increases blood circulation to the brain and re-energizes the entire body.

THE HEADSTAND

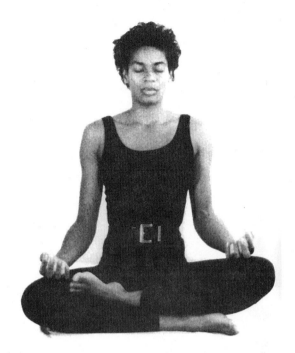

THE CROSS-LEGGED POSTURE

THE CROSS-LEGGED POSTURE

(SUKHASANA)

Sit in a cross-legged position. Keep the head and trunk straight. Place the feet beneath the knees. Place your hands on your thighs.

An easy meditative posture, it increases the blood supply in the pelvic region. It decreases the respiration and metabolic rates. The focus point is on breathing.

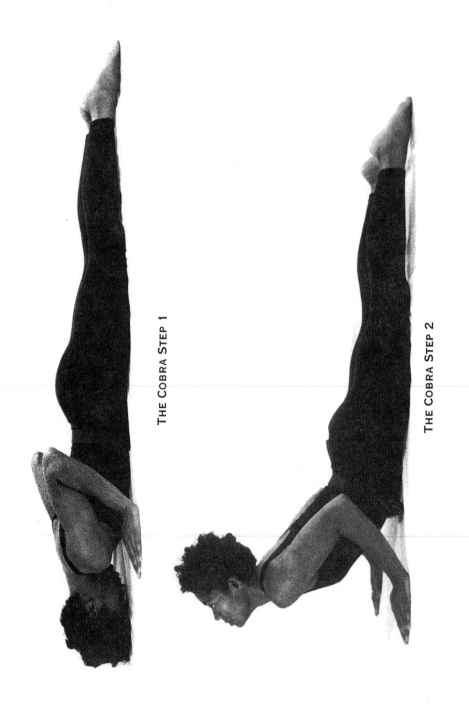

THE COBRA STEP 1

THE COBRA STEP 2

THE COBRA

(BHUJANGASANA)

Lie on your stomach, placing your forehead on the floor with arms at your sides. Inhale. Slowly raise your head, stretching forward and upward, then also slowly raise the shoulders. Hold this position for several deep breaths. Then bend your elbows, placing your hands besides your chest at shoulder level. Continue to raise your chest with the arms balancing the body. Do not raise your stomach off the floor. Breathe evenly. Maintain this position for several deep breaths, then exhale slowly while lowering your body and finally placing your forehead on the floor. Repeat this sequence three times. Finally, bring your arms against the body and relax.

The cobra affects the sympathetic nervous system and the nervous system as a whole. The muscles of the shoulders, neck, and back, flexibility of the spine, elasticity of the lungs, and circulation around the vertebrae are also all enhanced. The focus point is on the spine and back.

THE SCALE

(MAYOORASANA)

Assume a kneeling position on the floor with knees apart. Bend forward, place the palms on the floor with fingers pointed towards the feet. Bend your elbows and rest your stomach on the elbows and your chest on your upper arms. Extend your legs. Exhale. Hold your body weight on your hands. Raise your legs up and your trunk and head forward. The body is parallel to the floor. Hold the posture for several deep breaths.

This posture tones the abdominal area. Blood circulation and abdominal organs functions are enhanced. Stimulates digestive function. Because of the pressure of the elbows on the stomach, the abdominal aorta is partially compressed and the blood is directed toward the digestive organs. The live, pancreas, stomach, and kidneys are toned. The intra-abdominal pressure is increased which tone the abdominal viscera. The focus point is on balance.

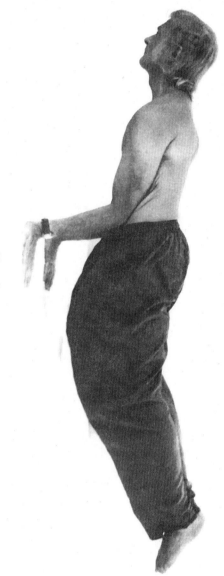

THE SCALE

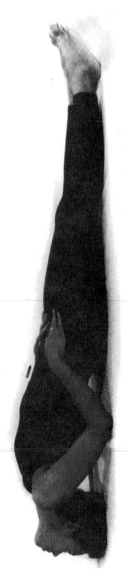

THE FISH

THE FISH

(MATSYASANA)

Lie on your back with arms at your sides. Inhale. Arch the back, tilt your head back, and place the crown of the head on the floor. Use your forearms and elbows to help support you. Expand your chest. Breathe evenly. Maintain this position for several deep breaths, then slowly come back to the starting position.

The Fish affects the cervical vertebrae, neck, solar plexus, thyroid gland, and the skin.

The focus point is on the thyroid gland.

THE KNEELING POSTURE
(VAJRASANA)

Sit in a kneeling position. Keep the head and trunk straight. Place the hands on the knees with palms facing down. Sit on your inner soles, toes touching, with heels pointed out. If you do not feel comfortable sit on the floor just touching your buttocks with your feet. The Kneeling Posture tones the pelvic area and improves digestion. The focus point is on breathing

    The cross-legged and kneeling posture is suitable for breathing exercises, concentration, and meditation if the Half-Lotus or Lotus postures are uncomfortable for you.

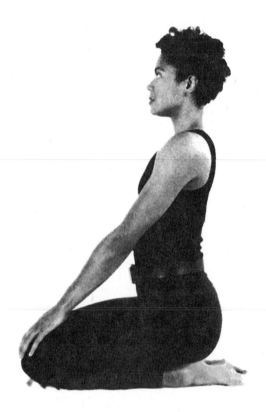

THE KNEELING POSTURE

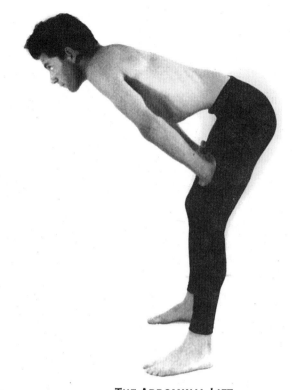

THE ABDOMINAL LIFT

THE ABDOMINAL LIFT
(UDDIYANA BANDHA)

The abdominal lift has entire body effect and provides a natural "massage" to the stomach, colon, intestines, gallbladder and pancreas. It also affects the visceral organs and glands. The focus point is on the navel center.

Stand with feet apart, knees bent slightly and pointing outward, hands on the upper thighs. Lower the trunk, but do not bend the trunk forward. Exhale deeply, forcibly. Now imagine that you are going to take a deep breath, but do not inhale. "Suck" the abdomen inward and upward the abdomen. The intestines and the naval are drawn toward the back. But do not inhale. Only the abdominal muscles are working. The throat is closed. Hold the lift for a few seconds, then quickly and strongly push the abdomen out.

Start with 5 lifts per exhalation and increase up from 15-20 lifts per exhalation. The exhalation with its lifts constitutes one round. After terminating each round, inhale deeply and straighten up slowly; then relax for a few seconds and breathe normally.

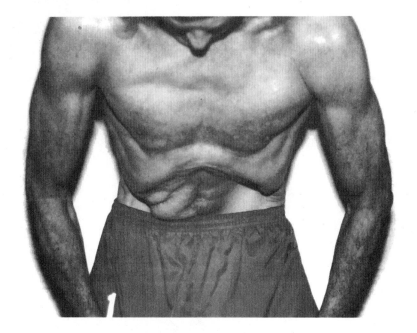

NAULI (A)

NAULI

Stand with your Legs apart, bent slightly at the knees. Put you hands on your thighs. Exhale and execute the abdominal lift (Uddiyana Bandha). Now contract the sides of the abdomen, (A) isolating the central abdomen muscle. Press on alternate hands to move the muscle from right to left. (B)

You can also rotate the central abdominal muscle in a churning motion. (C) This asana requires, control, manipulation and involuntary muscle use. This needs concentration and practice.

The focus point is on the abdomen. Nauli tones the stomach, intestines and live. It increase the flow of prana.

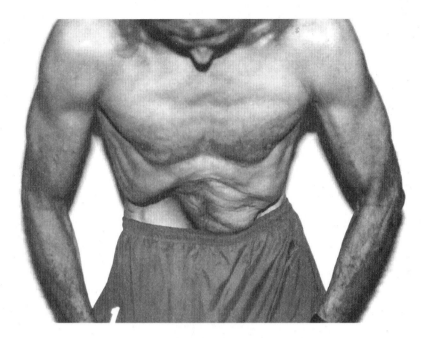

NAULI (B)

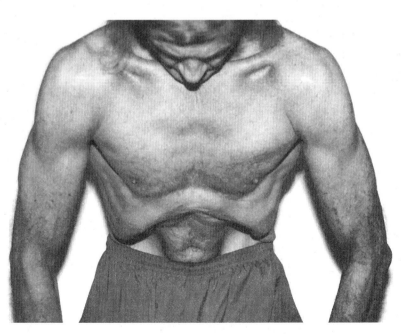

NAULI (C)

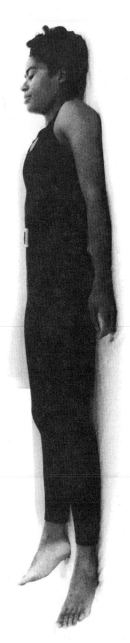

The Relaxation Posture

THE RELAXATION POSTURE
(SAVASANA)

This is one of the most important postures for compound or entire body effect. Lie on your back, arms beside the body, with palms facing up. Legs are slightly apart. Close your eyes. Let yourself go. Allow all your muscles to relax. The focus point is relaxation, total calmness, harmony, and peace.

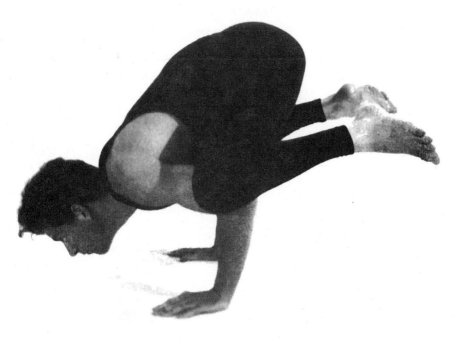

THE CROW

THE CROW

(KAKASANA)

Sit on your heels in a squat position, on your toes. Keep your knees apart. Put your palms firmly on the floor, parallel to your toes. Choose a point on the floor in front of you and focus on it. Place and rest your knees on your respective arms. Raise slowly from your toes, balancing your body on your arms. Maintain this position as long as you can. Repeat. The affects and focus point are the same as for the Side Crow.

THE SIDE CROW

(PARSWA KAKASANA)

In this variation, put the right thigh across the elbows of your arms and balance. Repeat the same exercise on the other side.

A more difficult variation of the side crow posture is when you slowly straighten the legs in the side crow posture.

The crow postures strengthen the arms, wrists, shoulders, improve balance, concentration, and breathing capacity (by expanding the chest).

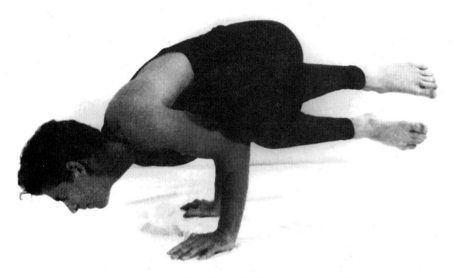

THE SIDE CROW

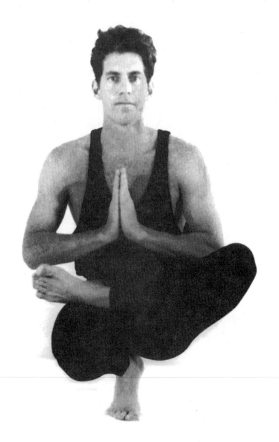

The Tiptoe Posture

The Tiptoe Posture
(Padandgushtasana)

Assume a kneeling position. Choose a spot and focus on it. Raise your knees slowly. Balance on your toes. Raise your right leg and put your foot over the left thigh. Hold a few seconds, then alternate to the other side. You can slowly raise up and down. This posture improves balance and concentration, regenerates the tired muscles of the feet and ankles. The focus point is on balance.

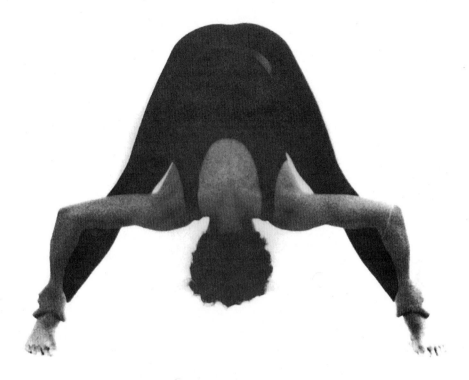

THE TRIANGLE "A"

THE TRIANGLE "A"
(PRASARITA PADOTTA-NASANA)

Stand with feet far apart and arms to the side at shoulder level. Inhale. Exhale. Bend forward slowly as far as you can, then grasp both ankles and pull gently. Try to get your body as close to the legs as possible. Hold for a few seconds. Relax, attune into the posture. Then relax, hang your arms loose, breath regularly and easily.

This posture improves flexibility,and stretches and strengthens the inner thighs and the ligaments and tendons of the legs. Improves digestion, circulation, and the function of the kidneys, spleen, and intestines. The focus point is on the hamstring and lower back.

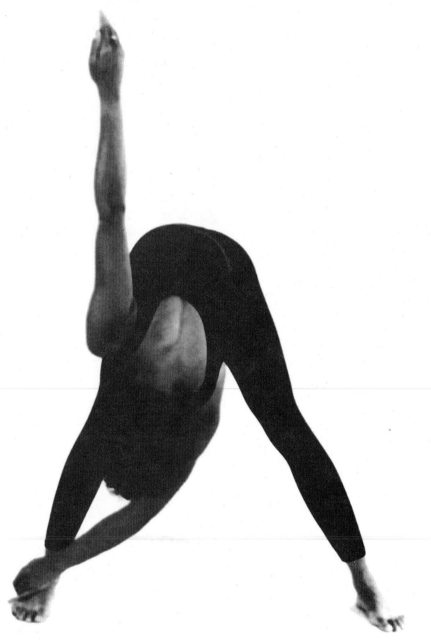

THE TRIANGLE WITH TWIST "B"

THE TRIANGLE WITH TWIST "B"
(PARIVRITTA TRIKONASANA)

Stand with feet far apart and arms to the side at shoulder level. Inhale. Exhale, bend forward, and simultaneously twist your torso downward. Grasp your right ankle with your left hand and pull gently as your right arm straightens up. Look at your left hand. Hold for a few seconds, then inhale and return to the starting position. Repeat to the other side.

Increases flexibility, tones the nerves of the spine, strengthens the hip joints. The focus point is on the hamstring.

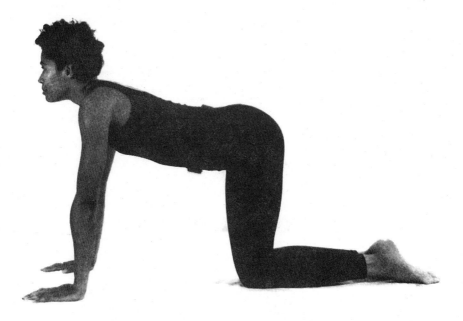

THE CAT STRETCH STEP 1

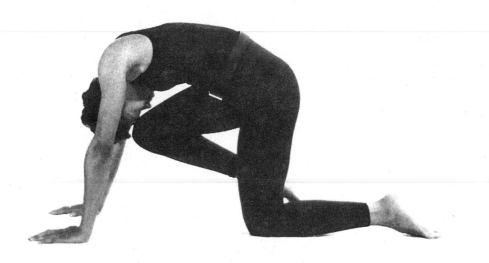

THE CAT STRETCH STEP 2

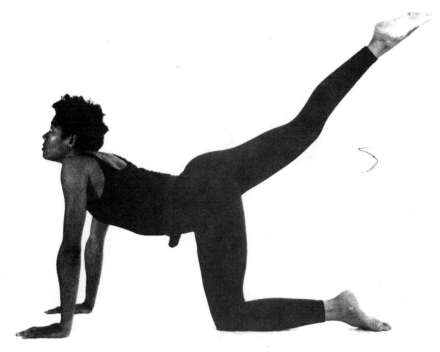

THE CAT STRETCH 3

THE CAT STRETCH

Assume a kneeling position on all fours, back parallel to the floor. Exhale, bend the left knee, lower the head, and bring the knee to the forehead. Hold this position for a few seconds. Inhale, extend and raise the leg and the head back as far as you can. Hold this position for a few seconds, then relax. Do the same with your right leg. Repeat 3-4 times. The Cat Stretch improves the actions of the intestines, heart, lungs, liver. It limbers the spinal column and relieves tension in the lower back. It also keeps the lower back limber and strengthens the legs, hip joints, shoulders. The focus point in on the lower back.

THE HEAD TO KNEE POSTURE
(JANU SIRASANA)

Assume a sitting position with your legs out in front of you. Bend your left leg and place your sole against your right inner thigh. Raise your arms up above your head. Inhale. Exhale and slowly bend forward as far as you can. Grasp your foot, ankle with both hands and bring your head down as far as you can. Hold this position for several deep breaths. Relax into the posture. Then slowly come back to the starting position. Repeat to the other side. The muscles of the back and the hamstrings are affected. Flexibility of the spine is increased. The focus point is the hamstring and back muscles.

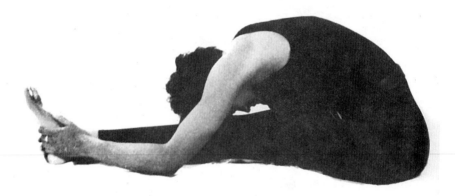

THE HEAD TO KNEE POSTURE

THE SHOULDER RAISE

Assume a kneeling position and sit on your heels, or a cross-legged position with your hands on your knees. Inhale and raise your shoulders up to the ears. Hold for a few seconds, then exhale and release the tension by dropping your shoulders. Repeat several times.

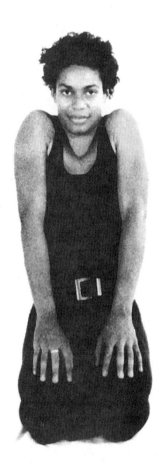

THE SHOULDER RAISE

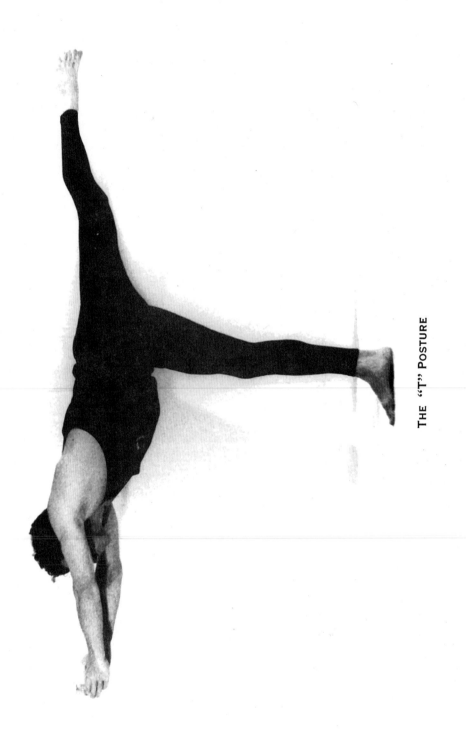

THE "T" POSTURE

THE "T" POSTURE

Assume a standing position with your arms over your head, hands together. Choose a spot and focus on it. Inhale. Exhale, bend your body forward parallel to the floor and raise your right leg up to the same level as your trunk to form a "T." The standing (left) leg is locked firmly. Hold for several seconds, then relax. Repeat with the opposite leg.

This posture develops balance, concentration, increases the flexibility of legs, hips, shoulders, and stretches the shoulders, hip, knee and ankle joints. The focus point is on balance.

THE BODY STRAIGHT POSTURE
(PADASANA)

Stand with legs together, hands parallel to shoulders, arms straight. Rise on your toes. Exhale, bend your arms and lower your body to the floor. Hold this position for a while. Inhale, extend your arms, "push up" tighten your abdominal, leg and arm muscles. Hold for a few seconds, then bend your arms, relax and lower your body to the floor. Repeat several times. This posture strengthens the wrists, arms, shoulders, back, and neck muscles. It improves circulation of the upper body. The focus point is the arms.

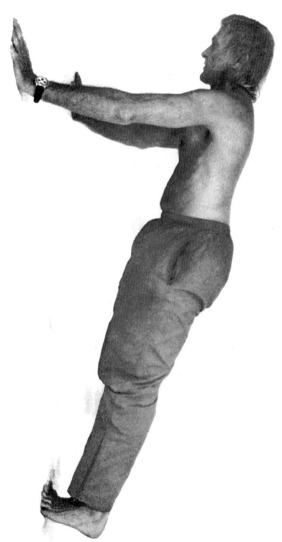

THE BODY STRAIGHT POSTURE

PADASANA VARIATION "A"

In this variation, simultaneously with the arm extension (push-up), raise your extended right leg high. Hold for a few seconds. Then exhale bend your arms relax and lower your body to the floor. Repeat with your left leg. The affects and focus point are the same as the Body Straight Posture.

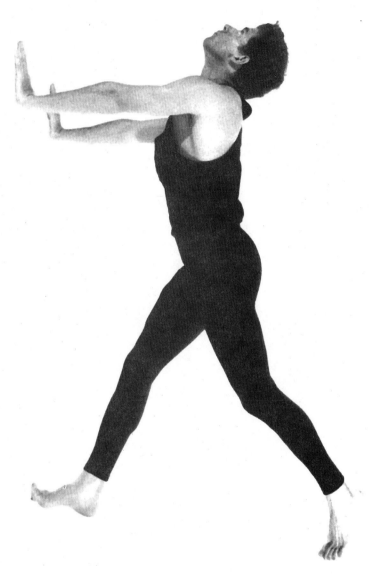

PADASANA VARIATION "A"

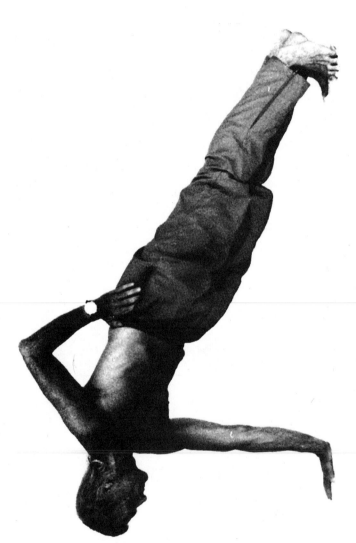

PADASANA VARIATION "B"

PADASANA VARIATION "B"

After push-up, raise the right arm behind the back. Extend the right leg straight out and parallel to the body to form a straight line. Hold this position. Repeat on other side.

PADASANA VARIATION "C"

The same as Padasana Variation "A" and "B" but each time as you bend your arms and lower your body to the floor, move both hands apart and then push-up (you can also move your hands forward to make the push-up more difficult).

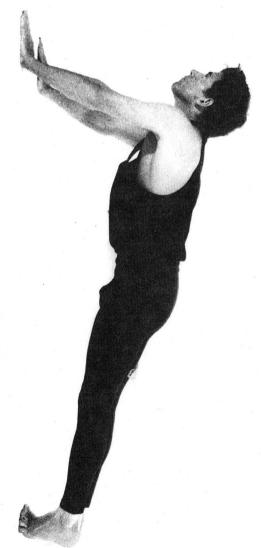

PADASANA VARIATION "C"

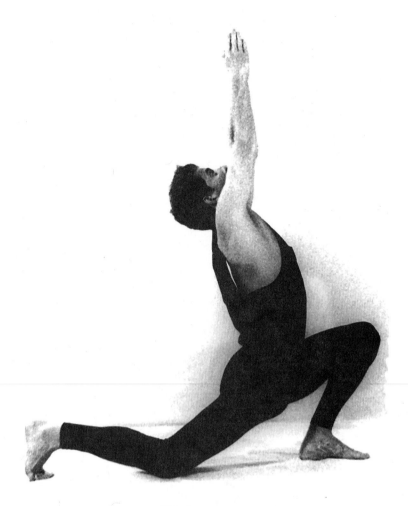

THE LUNGE

THE LUNGE

Assume a lunge position by stretching your right leg back as far as you can, keeping the right foot on the floor, bend the left knee, keeping it over the ankle. Inhale. Raise your arms above your head. Slowly bend back— arching the back as far as possible. Exhale, relax.

This posture stretches the pelvic muscles, the inner thighs, legs, and torso. The focus point is on the pelvic muscles.

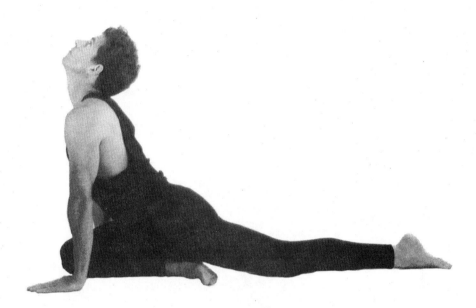

THE PIGEON POSTURE

THE PIGEON POSTURE
(MODIFIED RAJAKAPOTASANA)

Assume a kneeling position, sitting on your heels. Stretch your right leg back to a half "split" position keeping, your knee on the floor. Exhale, bend your trunk forward with your chest on your thigh and your forehead on the floor. Inhale;, raise your head, then your trunk up slowly as far as you can. Hold this position for several seconds. Then go back slowly to the starting position in a reverse order. Repeat 2-3 times.

This position has an all-over affect. It strengthens, stretches, and tones the spinal column, stretches the chest and rib cage, strengthens and stretches the muscles of the groin and hip joints as well as around the spinal column. It also stimulates the nerves around the spine assisting the metabolism and especially the reproductive glands and organs. The focus point is on the cervical and sacral vertebrae,

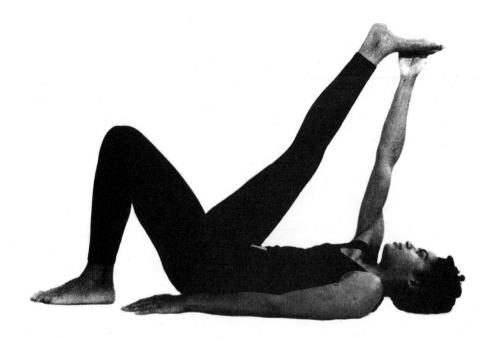

The Leg Stretch

The Leg stretch
(Supta Padangusthasana)

Lie on your back with your arms at your sides. Bend both knees. Now grasp your right foot with your right hand and raise the leg fully extended. If you can, also fully extend your left leg, keeping it firmly on the floor. Hold the stretch for several seconds. Return to the starting position. Repeat with your left leg. This position gives a deep stretch to the leg muscles and rejuvenates the muscles and nerves in the pelvis and hips. The focus point is on the stretching and rejuvenating of the muscles.

THE STANDING LEG STRETCH

Assume a standing position. Choose a spot in front of you and focus on it. Bend and raise your right knee. Grasp your foot with both hands, and slowly extend your leg forward and up. Bend your elbows close to your leg. Bend your head slowly and bring it to your knee. Hold this position for several seconds, Keep the standing leg straight, firmly on the floor. Then relax and repeat with your left leg. The affects and focus points are similar to the preceding asana, except this also works on balance.

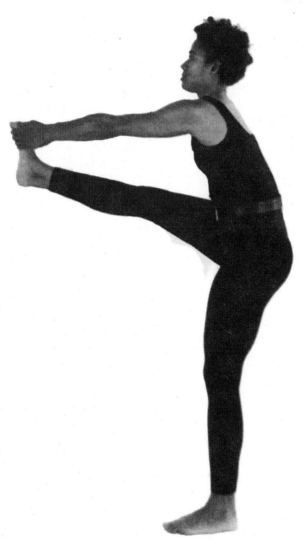

THE STANDING LEG STRETCH

YOGA SIT-UP

Sit with knees bent, trunk and head straight, arms outstretched at shoulder level. Slowly lie backward so as to be on your back, keeping arms in the original position.

Lift your chin toward your chest and slowly lift your shoulders and trunk as to make a sit-up, returning to the starting position. Repeat several times. You can increase the effect of the exercise by crossing your hands on your chest or behind your neck.

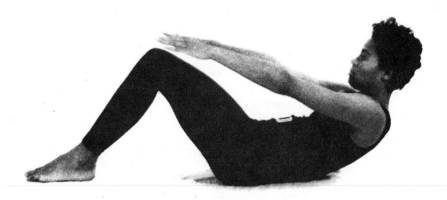

YOGA SIT-UP STEP 1

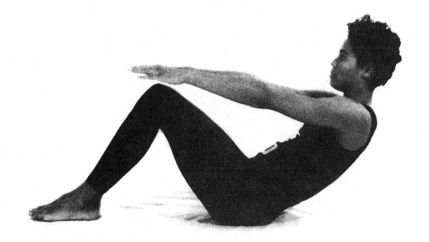

YOGA SIT-UP STEP 2

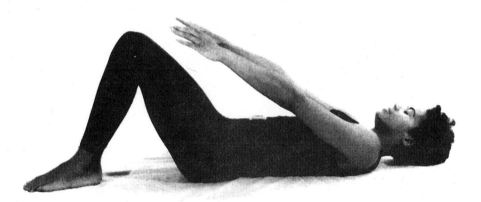

YOGA SIT-UP STEP 3

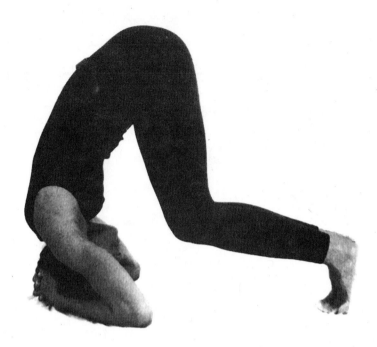

THE HALF HEADSTAND

THE HALF HEADSTAND

Assume a kneeling posture and sit on your heels. Interlock your fingers and place your elbows on the floor so that the elbows and the interlocked fingers form a triangle on the ground. Raise the hips slightly and place the head on the floor. Your interlocked fingers support the back of the head. Now straighten the legs and move your feet slightly forward until the back is perpendicular to the floor. Hold for several deep breaths, then release. This asana has similar affects has the full headstand position. In this variation, the cervical and thoracic parts of the vertical column get more pressure. The vertebral column is strengthened. The focus is on stretching the ligaments and muscles of the neck.

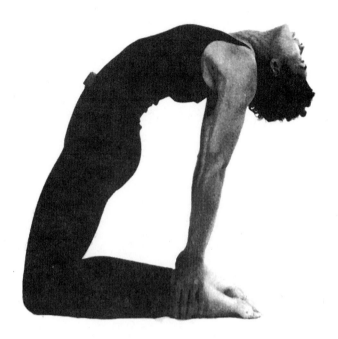

THE MODIFIED CAMEL

THE MODIFIED CAMEL POSTURE

Assume a kneeling position with your feet slightly apart, sitting on your heels. Grasp your ankles, inhale, arch (lift) your back and hips up and hold for several deep breaths. Breathe deeply. Come down slowly, and sit on your heels. Bend forward while exhaling and bring your arms above the head on the floor and stretch out. Relax.

This asana stretches the upper and lower thigh and knees. It limbers the entire spine and pelvis, opens the chest, and improves respiration. The focus point is on the spine.

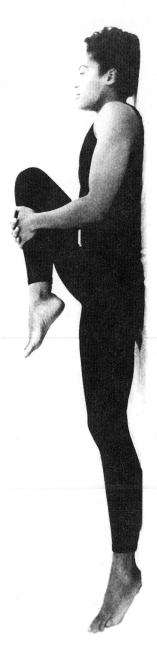

THE SINGLE KNEE SQUEEZE

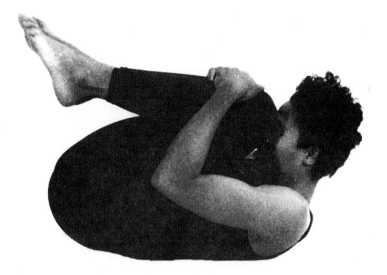

THE DOUBLE KNEE SQUEEZE

THE KNEE SQUEEZE

Lay flat on the floor. Bend your right knee and slowly bring it up to your chest. Grasp your knee with both hands and slowly pull it to your chest. The left leg remains on the floor. Feel the stretch in your lower back and in the left hip. Then repeat with the left leg, then with both legs. Repeat each exercise four times.

THE BRIDGE POSTURE

Lie on your back. Bend your knees. With feet flat on the floor and heels close to your buttocks, bring your arms above your head on the floor. Inhale and arch your back, lifting your hips up. Hold for several deep breaths, then exhale and come down slowly. Repeat 2-3 times. Then sit with your legs stretched out in front of you. Inhale and bring your arms above your head. Interlock your fingers and stretch your arms up. Hold for 2-3 seconds, then execute the Seated Forward Bend Posture. (Page 69)

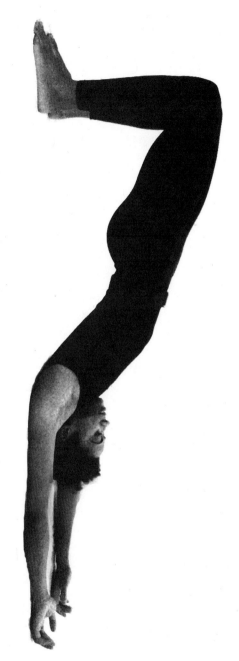

THE BRIDGE

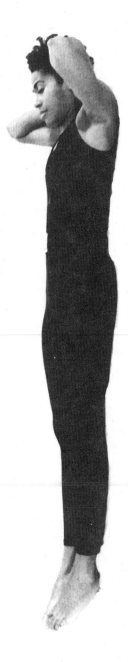

Neck Stretch

NECK STRETCH

Lie on your back. Interlace your fingers behind your neck. Exhale and pull your head up with the help of your arms, stretching up and pressing elbows together. Hold this position for several deep breath. Inhale and slowly lower the head to the starting position, arms placed beside the body, and release. The focus point is on the neck muscles.

SUMMARY

Yoga asanas have multiple effects. The same asana can be used for regeneration of strength, as well as for compensation of the muscle dysbalances produced by one-sided loading. It can also be used as a supplemental exercise. The same asana can be used for practicing concentration, or for warm-up and cool-down. What asana you select depends on your particular needs and goals, and when you practice it. For example, you can incorporate the Standing Forward Bend Posture, with the focus point on relaxation (for a psychological affect) in your cool-down exercises for the purpose of regeneration after your training session. If you choose the same asana for improving concentration and/or for warm-up with the focus point on the hamstring and back muscles, you will gain a physiological affect.

Now that you are aware of the technique and effects of yoga postures, you will be able to determine the appropriate asanas to incorporate into your training schedule based on analysis of your needs and of your sport.

In the following section, you will find examples of yoga regimens constructed by athletes for various purposes as part of their sport training.

PART III

THE REGIMENS

6 ━━━━

REGIMENS USED BY TOP ATHLETES

Keep in mind that yoga asanas can be combined into batteries for specific purposes. Examples:

SUPPLEMENTAL EXERCISE FOR ATHLETES

What follows is a battery of supplemental exercises for home practice. The advantages of this battery, as with all yoga asanas, is low demand on space, time, and equipment. This battery positively affects the mental state, the process of recovery (regeneration), improves the elasticity of the spine, relaxes the muscles, and benefits the cardiovascular system and other organs and body functions. Practice the asanas in the following order:

- The Cross-legged (Meditative) posture (Page 73)

  Breathe slowly and deeply. Concentrate on your breathing, for 2-3 minutes. Feel your belly moving in and out.
- Modified Sitting Forward Bend (Page 50)
- The Cobra (Page 74)
- The Bow (Page 68)
- The Shoulderstand (Page 67)
- The Plough (Page 71)
- The Fish (Page 78)
- The Twisting Position (Page 51)
- The Relaxation Posture (Page 84)

WARM-UP ASANA BATTERY

Using yoga during warm-up serves two functions: it is a means for practicing attention and concentration, and it helps warm-up the muscles. You can simultaneously improve your flexibility, body awareness, and self-control. Although these yoga exercises take only 2-3 minutes, you will find them very useful in shifting yourself from a usual state of awareness into a more concentrated state. After finishing your concentration exercises, continue with your regular warm-up routine.

Start each training and competition with sitting still and concentrating for 2-3 minutes on breathing. This brief exercise will be a mental tune-up for you.

After this short term concentration/meditation exercise, start your regular warm-up routine. However, for the first one or two exercises of your warm-up regimen, choose a yoga posture which you should execute with total (passive) concentration. Two good postures to use for this are the foreward bend and the seated foreward bend (See Pages 38 and 46). The focal point during both yoga postures is on the hamstring and on the muscles of the back (the physiological effect of the postures).

Through yoga, concentration becomes as much a part of the warm-up routine as the daily stretching. Like physical exercises, practicing concentration becomes a habit when done regularly and systematically.

YRE FOR SHORT TERM REST

Yoga is an excellent tool for relaxing and regenerating muscles between training sessions or competition when a complete cool-down is not needed (for example,between the bouts, heats, etc.). After completing a training session or following a competition or at other times when short rest is needed, lie on your back (savasana) and allow all your body to rest, breathing easily. Each time you exhale, mentally repeat the word "calm." Maintain this position for 30-60 seconds, then assume the following position:

MODIFIED FISH

Lying on your back, cross your legs and place your hands below your head. Now inhale deeply and then very slowly exhale. Breathe through your nose. Exhale all the air very slowly. Then pause for 2-3 seconds before inhaling again. Now inhale fully. When you inhale, visualize and feel cold air going through your nostrils; when exhaling visualize and feel the warm air leaving your nostrils. Practice this for 1-3 minutes.

After completing this exercise, maintain the Relaxation Posture (Page 78) for a little while longer, repeating the word "calm" each time you exhale. Then gradually reactivate the muscles of the whole body by tensing, then standing.

In this Modified Fish posture, the dorsal back region is fully extended and the chest is fully expanded. Breathing will become fuller. This position enables relaxation of the arteries and veins that transport blood to the heart and back. The expanded rib cage allows for a more effective workout.

This technique produces calmness and a refreshing physical sensation that stimulates overall recovery.

YOGA BATTERY OF ASANAS FOR COOL-DOWN

As in the warm-up routine, at the end of each training and competition choose two to four yoga asanas for speeding up the process of regeneration and practicing concentration. For example, B. Atkins, NCAA champion in foil and epee fencing, uses the following YRE in his cool-down:

- The Modified Standing Forward Bend (Page 40)
- The Seated Forward Bend (Page 69)
- The Half Lotus (Page 61)
- The Modified Cobra (Page 44)
- The Half Plough (Page 42)
- The Relaxation Posture (Page 84)

ASANAS TO PREVENT, REHABILITATE BACK PAIN

This battery consists of selected and modified yoga asanas for both strengthening the abdominal and hip extensor muscles and stretching the lower back and hip flexor muscles.

- Yoga Sit-up (Page 110-111)
- The Knee Squeeze (Page 114-115)
- The Locust (Page 47)
- The Half Plough (Page 42)
- The Modified Half Locust (Page 48)
  Raise the leg bent at the knee about 90 degrees.
- The Twist (Page 52)

ASANAS FOR RELAXING TIRED LEGS AFTER INTENSIVE WORKOUT

The following battery of yoga asanas speeds up the process of regeneration (elimination of the products of fatigue) by applying pull, rotation, pressure, and the force of gravity. This increases the flexibility, and elasticity of the leg muscles and ligaments.

Select a few, or practice all the presented asanas according to your needs. Maintain the final position (focus point) for several deep breaths, then relax. Finish the selected battery with the savasana (relaxation posture).

- Modified Standing Forward Bend (Page 40)
  Maintain the final position for several deep breaths.
- The Half-Lotus (Page 61)
- The Groin Stretch (Page 60)
- The Shoulderstand (Page 67)
- The Triangle (Pages 89-90)
- The Leg Stretch (Page 108)
- The Standing Leg Stretch (Page 109)
- The Resting Posture (Page 64)

- The Frog (Page 56)

  Maintain for several deep breaths. Relax in a comfortable standing position.

- The Eagle Posture (Page 57)

- Maintain for several deep breaths. Alternate legs. Relax when standing up. Shake your legs to loosen them.

- The Relaxation Posture (Page 84)

  Relax for several deep breaths.

YRE FOR RELEASING SHOULDER TENSION

Athletes are aware that shoulder tension can have a disastrous effect on the execution of many sport skills. For example, shoulder tension will cause an unsuccessful riposte in fencing, a bad serve in tennis, an unsuccessful freethrow in basketball, etc.

When we are under pressure, stress automatically contracts the muscles of the shoulders. Stress, anxiety,and emotions as well as fatigue after hard training all produce shoulder tension. The following battery of YRE will help you release the shoulder tension:

- The Shoulder Raise (Page 95)
- The Modified Chest Expansion (Page 66)
- The Bridge Posture (Page 117)
- The Modified Camel Posture (Page 113)
- The Modified Bow Posture (Page 54)
- The Seated Forward Bend (Page 69)

YRE FOR RELEASING NECK TENSION

Like shoulder tension, neck tension can be the product of hard training, stress, pressure, and mental or emotional tensions. Use the following YRE for releasing neck tension:

- Assume a cross-legged position. Exhale and slowly bend your head forward to stretch the neck muscles. Hold for several deep breath, then inhale and slowly tilt your head back.

Hold again this position for several deep breath. Repeat 3-4 times. Then turn your head slowly to the right and hold this position for several deep breaths, then slowly turn your head to the left side. Keep your trunk and shoulders straight during the exercise. Repeat it 3-4 times.

- The Half Headstand (Page 112)
- The Neck Stretch (Page 118)
- The Fish (Page 78)

Because shoulder and neck tension usually occur simultaneously, it is useful to combine this battery with YRE for releasing shoulder tension.

YRE FOR RAPID RELEASE OF BODY TENSION

Body tension can be developed by fatigue after hard training, by stress, emotions, etc. The modified bow posture stimulates the solar plexus, blood circulation and functions of the organs in the stomach cavity. It also strengthens the lower back muscles, increases intra-abdominal pressure and promotes increased blood supply to the internal organs.

- The Modified Bow (Page 54)
- The Half Plough (Page 42)

    Lie on your back and execute the posture with knees slightly bent, to stretch the muscles of your back. Hold this position for several deep breaths. Then come back to the starting position.

- The Relaxation Posture (Page 84)

YRE FOR RELEASING TENSION IN THE DIAPHRAGM, ABDOMINAL MUSCLES AND STIMULATING AND STRENGTHENING THE FUNCTIONS OF DIGESTIVE ORGANS

Tension in the abdominal muscles and diaphragm causes misfunctioning of the digestive organs leading to digestion problems. The following battery of YRE releases the abdominal tension and strengthens the functions of digestive organs:

- The Knee Bending Posture

  Stand straight, feet together, arms on the waist. Choose a spot and focus on it. Inhale and rise onto your toes. Exhale slowly. Bend slowly at your knees. Maintain this position for a few seconds, then slowly come back to the starting position. Relax.

- Double Knee Squeeze (Page 115)
- The Bow (Page 68)

SALUTATION TO THE SUN

This battery of asana is executed continuously. The battery has a complete (entire body) effect. All the plexuses of the body, the circulatory, pulmonary, nervous systems, digestive organs and big muscle groups are affected. It affects each sequence of the spine and all joints. It is most useful in stretching and warming-up the muscles and joints and for loading the cardiovascular system. Controlled breathing is applied.

1. Stand straight with arms bent at elbow, hands together in a "prayer" position.
2. Lean backward (stretching) while raising your arms over your head. Inhale.
3. Bend forward and touch the floor with your hands (knees are extended but not locked). Exhale.
4. Bring your left foot back to a lunge position while bending the right knee. Inhale.
5. Bring your right foot back next to the left foot to a "push-up" position. Hold your breath.
6. Lower your body down, raise your elbows, and rest on your hands. The hands, chin, knees and toes are on the floor, the stomach is raised above the floor. Exhale.
7. Assume the cobra position. Extend your arms, raise your head, shoulders, and chest. The rest of the body is flat on the floor. Inhale.
8. Raise your body to form a high peak with your buttocks (This is also called the downward dog position). Exhale.

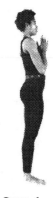

STEP 1

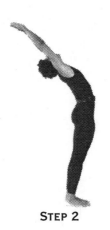

STEP 2

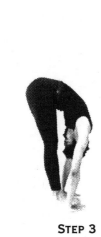

STEP 3

STEP 4

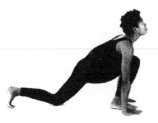

STEP 5

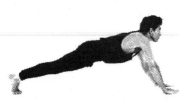

STEP 6

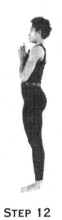

STEP 12

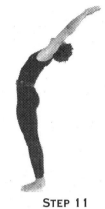

STEP 11

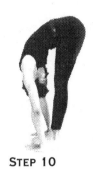

STEP 10

STEP 9

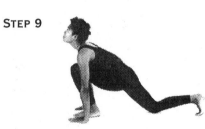

STEP 8

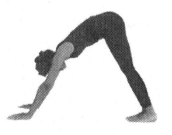

STEP 7

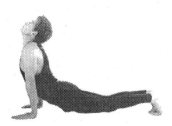

9. Assume the lunge position as in step number 4 by bringing your left foot forward between your arms. Inhale.

10. Repeat step 3. Exhale.

11. Repeat step 2. Inhale.

12. Repeat step 1.

The effect of this routine, called the Sun Salutation, or Surya Namaskar, is increased by the number of repetitions of the battery. Repeating the routine up to 30-50 times is excellent loading for the cardiovascular system as well as for the muscles. If you execute these movements slowly, they have a calming, deactivating effect. If you execute them fast, repeating the series 8-10 times with full inhalation, it has a stimulating, activating effect on the nervous system.

SALUTATION TO THE MOON

This battery (similar to the previous one) has 13 postures which are executed with controlled breathing. The battery has a calming, balancing effect on the physical and mental state.

1. Stand straight, with arms bent at elbow, hands together in a "prayer" position.

2. Lean backward (stretching) while simultaneously raising arms over the head. Inhale.

3. Bend forward and touch the floor with your hands (knees are extended but not locked). Exhale.

4. Bring your left foot back to a lunge position while bending the right knee. Inhale.

5. Bring your right foot back next to the left foot to a "push-up" position. Hold your breath.

6. Bring your knees to the floor sliding your hands back and stretch back. The hips touch the buttocks. Exhale.

7. Bend your knees and elbows. The chin, chest and knees are on the floor. Exhale.

8. Assume the "cobra" position. Raise your head, shoulders and chest. Rest on your hands. The rest of the body is flat on the floor. Inhale.

9. Slide your hands back and raise your body to form a high peak with your buttocks (downward dog). Exhale then inhale.

10. Repeat step 6. Exhale.

11. Repeat step 4. Inhale.

12. Stand and repeat step 2.

13. Repeat step 1.

Execute the battery of asanas very slowly with deep, slow inhalations and exhalations. The battery has a calming effect. Complete 3-5 repetitions.

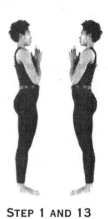

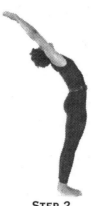

STEP 2

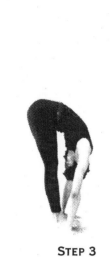

STEP 3

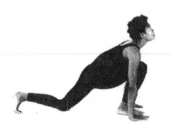

STEP 4

STEP 5

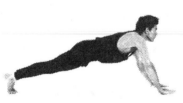

STEP 6

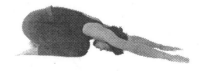

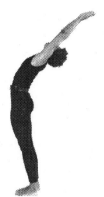

STEP 12

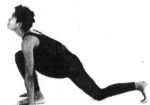
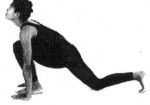

STEP 11

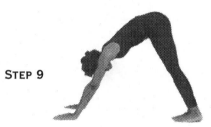
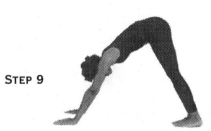

STEP 10

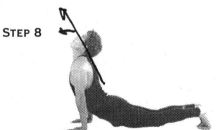

STEP 9

STEP 8

STEP 7

EXAMPLE OF ATHLETE'S TOTAL YOGA TRAINING

- The Cross-legged Posture with meditation for 3-5 minutes (Page 73)
- The Seated Forward Bend (Page 69)
- The Cobra (Page 74)
- The Locust or The Half Locust (Page 47-48)
- The Bow (Page 68)
- The Plough (Page 71)
- The Twist (Page 52)
- The Shoulderstand (Page 67)
- The Fish (Page 78)
- The Abdominal Lift (Page 81)
- Meditative sit with breathing exercises "sitting still" – detachment, concentration (meditation) (Page 60 or 61)
- The Relaxation Posture (Page 84)
- Reactivation including taking a few deep breaths, sitting (standing) up, exercising with the arms, and mentally repeating the autosuggestive phrases: "*the sensation of heaviness is disappearing from my arms and legs. I feel refreshed, reenergized, and fully alert.*"

THE "DOUBLE R" BREATH FOR FOCUSING IN CASE OF HIGH STRESS

During competition, when pressure is high, when you have lost your focus, when your confidence has decreased, when you doubt yourself, have negative thoughts, etc., use the yoga technique which I call "Double R" breath.

- Take a deep slow inhalation and focus your attention on the image that with this yoga breath you "recharge," accumulate your energy (prana), your life force. Each cell of your body is supplied with an extra amount of energy and life force.

- Slowly exhale and focus your attention on releasing the tension of the muscles of your neck, shoulders, trunk, and legs in the mentioned order. Visualize that with releasing the muscle tension simultaneously you decrease the negative emotions.

My students use this "Double R" technique successfully between fencing bouts, or when they are confused or tense, They claim it helps them to "re-focus," to "get back on the track." Some of my students, when they are confused, take a "tactical break" during the bout to use the double "R" technique to regain the focus and mental balance. Mind is the master of the senses, and breath is the master of the mind.

RHYTHMIC YOGA BREATHING WHEN WALKING

- Walk with your trunk and head straight.
- Inhale slowly, counting in your mind 1, 2, 3, 4. One count to each step (diaphragmatic yoga breath).
- Exhale slowly, deeply through your nostrils during steps 8.
- Later you can prolong your breathing for 6-8 counts (steps).

When you feel your excitement or stress level is too high before starting the performance, or during the breaks, you can use the complete yoga breathing to decrease the level of arousal, to re-focus, or to clear your mind. You can achieve this effect, also with the complet yoga breath and alternate nostril breathing.

THE TENSION RELEASING BREATH

- Take a complete yoga inhalation. Retain the breath for a few seconds.

- Exhale slowly throw your mouth with your lips puckered as if to whistle; exhale a little air, then stop for a moment, retaining the air, and then contine exhaling.

- The exhalations should be done with vigor. Repeat these steps several times. As you exhale, visualize releasing the tension and emotions.

This technique quiets the mind and releases tension and negative emotions. When you are tired, you will find this breathing refreshes the nervous system. My fencers used this technique for releasing the tension and emotions during the bouts and during short pauses. Complete yoga breathing recharges your energy, and is a unique way to re-energize the brain cells or pick up your energy as it lags during the course of the day.

BATTERY OF ASANAS FOR IMPROVING BALANCE AND CONCENTRATION

The following asanas develop balance and concentration, besides many other benefits. When assuming one of the balance postures, first choose a focus point to gaze at. This will facilitate assuming and balancing the posture. You will find that if your mind wanders or you lose the focus, you lose your balance also. Incorporate one or two asanas into your daily training regimen, both for improving the sense of balance and concentration.

- The Tree Posture (Page 53)
- The Dancer's Posture (Page 58)
- The Scale (Page 77)
- The Crow (Page 86)
- The Side Crow (Page 87)
- The "T" Posture (Page 96)
- The Knee Bending Posture (Page 129)
- The Tiptoe Posture (Page 88)

- The Standing Leg Stretch (Page 109)
- The Eagle Posture (Page 57)

Using Yoga As Supplemental Training

Yoga is suitable for supplemental training because of its many-sided effects. Among the goals of practicing a supplemental training program such as yoga is to maintain a healthy balance in the body by compensating for the one-sided system of exercises typical in any given sport. By practicing yoga with its set of movements and exercises, an athlete can achieve this balance. The task of yoga supplemental exercises is also to develop those muscle groups that are not directly used in the regular practice. Not only does this increase performance, but it also helps maintain health for the athlete. The athlete can practice the yoga asanas anytime and anywhere without the need for special equipment or workout space.

Yoga also helps decrease the negative effects of a sports training program. These negative effects include small deformations which, over a long period of time, can damage the body or can lead to the development of improper body posture. Prevention of injury and yoga as a supplemental sport training program go hand in hand.

In the following pages you will find examples of using yoga exercises for compensation of the one-sided effects of training in different sports.

I suggest including the following exercises in all sports preparation:

- Abdominal breathing, complete yoga breath, althernate nostril breathing, the double "R" breath.
- Exercises of the four basic steps—body awareness, breath awarenss, attention focus and concentration.
- YRE, YSE
- Transcendental mediation or Autogenic Training

BOXING

Boxing has a many-sided effect on the body, effectively developing the respiratory system in addition to strength. However, supplemental exercises are useful to assure optimum health. A complete yoga training with focus on asanas effecting the spine as well as asanas developing a sense of balance are recommended. Also, the practice of Raja Yoga optimizes reaction time, and especially, facilitates the combination of punch and quick decision making.

Suggested exercises:

- YRE for speeding up the recovery process
- Yoga breathing exercises—abdominal breathing, complete yoga breath, alternate nostril breathing, the double "R" breath
- Suppplemental exercise for athletes
- The Abdominal Lift
- The Nauli
- TM, AT

Suggested supplemental exercises are:

- Complete yoga training as supplemental training (see Example of Athlete's Total Yoga Training on Page 130).
- Asanas affecting the spine and developing a sense of balance such as: The Cobra (Page 74), the Bow (Page 68), the Triangle (Pages 89-90), the Twist (Page 52), the Locust (Page 47), the Plough (Page 71), the Crow (Page 86), the Scale (Page 77).
- YRE relaxing tired legs after intensive loading. (Page 126)
- Yoga breathing exercises: Abdominal and rhythmic yoga breathing. (Page 137-138)
- Raja Yoga exercises for controlling the mental and emotional states.

BIKING

From the point of view of health, biking has similar effects on the body as skating. In addition, heavy pressure is put on the circulatory system, making breathing more difficult. The position of the body during biking interferes with the intercoastal (middle) breathing, however, diaphragmatic breathing is well developed. The insufficient intercoastal breathing negatively affects the blood circulation in the rib cage which further loads the right side of the heart. Also, the dusty environment of the roads negatively effects the respiratory system.

Complete yoga breathing exercises, with emphasis on the intercoastal and clavicula phases, is recommended to balance breathing. Also, those asanas that invert the body will move blood into the upper half of the body, compensating for the concentration of blood circulation in the lower extremities due to the emphasis on the lower extremities during training. They will also help prevent, in men, inflammation of the prostrate due to long periods of sitting.

Permanent loading of the leg muscles negatively affects the blood circulation of capillaries due to lack of total relaxation of muscles between the single contraction of muscles. This can contribute to arthritis. Biking develops deformation of the spine (kyphosis of the lower vertebras). Asanas which effect the spine should be practiced. Bicyclists need to work with asanas that will flex the spine in the opposite direction and reverse circulation.

For bicyclists, the suggested exercises are:

- The Cobra (Page 74), the Bow (Page 68), the Triangle (Page 89-90), the Modified Cobra (Page 44), the Modified Bow (Page 54), the Twist (Page 52), the Cat Stretch (Pages 92-93), the Pigeon Posture (Page 107), the Modified Camel Posture (Page 113) the Locust (Page 47) the "T" Posture (Page 96).
- To reverse blood flow: The Shoulderstand (Page 67), the Half Shoulderstand (Page 43), the Headstand (Page 72).
- Yoga breathing exercises: The abdominal and rhythmic yoga breathing (Page 137-138).

- YRE for speeding up the recovery process after hard training and competition (Page 126).

- Practicing autogenic training for withstanding the rigors of the intensive training (see Chapters 14 and 15).

- Raja Yoga exercises for controlling the mental and emotional states and for developing concentration.

FENCING

Fencing develops fast reflexive coordination of muscle actions to such a high degree that fencing can be considered a "sport of the nervous system." Fencing is a "one-sided sport" and, therefore, requires broad supplemental training. For fencers, the suggested exercises are:

- Complete yoga training as supplemental and compensational training (see examples of athlete's total yoga training on Page 136).

- Raja Yoga exercises for speeding up the reflexes, the process of analysis of the bout situation, and decision making.

- Raja Yoga exercises for controlling the mental and emotional states, and for developing concentration.

- YRE for speeding up the recovery process after hard training and competition (Page 126).

- Yoga breathing exercises, abdominal, and rhythmic breathing, the double "R" breathing (Page 137-138).

- Incorporate "sitting still steadily" and concentration on the breathing, the Modified Standing Forward Bend (Page 40), the Seated Forward Bend (Page 69) into your regular warm-up routine for both practicing concentration and for warm-up.

- Practicing autogenic training individually tailored for your specific needs.

GOLF

The big advantage of golf is the clean, healthy, outdoor environment. However, golf is also a one-sided sport (see Chapter 4). Here, also, complex yoga training is suggested as supplemental and compensational training.

The suggested exercises are:

- Complete yoga training as supplemental training (see Example of athletes total yoga training on page 136).
- Raja Yoga exercises for controlling the mental and emotional states and for developing concentration.
- Practicing autogenic training individually tailored for your specific needs.
- Yoga breathing exercises: abdominal breathing, rhythmic yoga breathing, the double "R" breath, complete yoga breathing when walking (Page 137-138).
- Asanas for improving the flexibility of the spine and asanas which strengthen the lower back.
- Battery of asanas for both rehabilitating the lower back, and prevention of pain and injury (Page 126).
- The Cobra (Pages 44, 74), the Triangle (Pages 89-90), the Twist (Page 52), the Dancer's Posture (Page 58).

GYMNASTICS (OLYMPIC)

This sport affects all muscles of the body. Therefore, asanas which develop the muscles of the trunk and abdomen would be useless for gymnasts. These athletes need to concentrate on asanas that affect the spine to prevent the development of so called "gymnastic back," a deformation of the spine.

For gymnasts, the suggested exercises are:

- The Cobra (Page 74), the Bow (Page 68), the Triangle (Pages 89-90), the Pigeon Posture (Page 107), the Modified Camel Posture (Page 113), the Twist (Page 52).
- Raja Yoga exercises for controlling the mental and emotional states and for developing concentration.
- YRE for speeding up the recovery process after hard training and competition (Page 126). Yoga breathing exercises: abdominal breathing, Complete and rhythmic yoga breathing (Page 137-138).

- Incorporate "sitting still steadily" and concentration on the breathing, and one or two yoga asanas into your regular warm-up routine for both practicing concentration and for warm-up.
- Practicing autogenic training for withstanding the rigors of the intensive training (see Chapters 14 and 15).

ICE SKATING, ICE HOCKEY, ROLLER SKATING

These sports do not have a complete effect on the development of the body. Therefore, yoga is a useful supplemental training. Skating requires a forward bend posture which interferes with proper breathing and blood circulation. The practice of yoga breathing exercises as a compensation exercise is recommended. Correct coordination of breathing with movement has positive effect on the body's thermoregulation system which, in turn, helps prevent the body from getting cold.

The suggested exercises are:

- YRE for speeding up the recovery process after hard training and competition (Page 126).
- Yoga breathing exercises: Abdominal and rhythmic yoga breathing, the double "R" breathing (Page 137-138).
- Practicing autogenic training for withstanding the rigors of the intensive training (see Chapters 14 and 15).
- Asana which effect the spine and strengthen the lower back. The Cobra (Pages 44, 74), the Bow (Pages 54, 68), the Triangle (Pages 89-90), the Twist (Page 52), the Locust (Page 47), the Pigeon Posture (Page 107), the Cat Stretch (Pages 92-93).
- Raja Yoga exercises for controlling the mental and emotional states.

SHOOTING, ARCHERY, YACHTING, RACE CAR DRIVING

These sports are also one-sided sports and have an uneven effect on the different organs of the body. Here, also, complex yoga training is suggested as supplemental and compensational training.

The suggested exercises are:

- Complete yoga training as supplemental training (see Example of athlete's total yoga training on Page 136).
- Raja Yoga exercises for controlling the mental and emotional states and for developing concentration.
- Practicing autogenic training individually tailored for your specific needs (Chapters 14 and 15)
- Yoga breathing exercises: abdominal breathing, and rhythmic yoga breathing, the double "R" breath, rhythmic yoga breathing when walking (Pages 137-138).

SKIING

From the point of view of health, cross-country skiing is one of the most valuable sports. The big advantage of skiing is the clean, healthy outdoor environment. Skiers need to concentrate on asanas which strengthen the lower back, and the knee joint and asanas which stretch the muscles of the legs.

The suggested exercises are:

- The Cobra (Pages 44, 74), the Triangle (Pages 89-90), the "T" posture (Page 96), the Pigeon Posture (Page 107), the Leg Stretch (108) the Standing Leg Stretch (Page 109), the Seated Forward Bend (Page 69), the Resting Posture (Page 64), battery of asanas for both rehabilitating the lower back, and prevention of pain and injury (Page 126).
- YRE for speeding up the recovery process after hard training and competition (Page 126).
- Yoga breathing exercises: Abdominal and rhythmic yoga breathing (Pages 137-138).

- Raja Yoga exercises for controlling the mental and emotional states and for developing concentration.
- Practicing autogenic training individually tailored for your specific needs (see Chapter 15).

SWIMMING, AQUATIC SPORTS

These are the most valuable sports from the aspect of yoga. In the water, the swimmer uses regulative, rhythmic breathing, just as in yoga. The pulmonary-respiratory system systems are effectively developed by swimming, water polo, and synchronized swimming. A big advantage of aquatic sports is the clean, healthy environment, free of dust.

For swimmers the suggested exercises are:

- YRE for speeding up the recovery process after hard training and competition (Page 126).
- Practicing autogenic training for withstanding the rigors of the intensive training (see Chapter 14).
- Yoga breathing exercises: Abdominal and rhythmic yoga breathing (Pages 137-138).
- Asanas for increasing the flexibility of the shoulder joints and asanas for stretching the lower back.
- The Triangle (Pages 89-90), the Cobra (Pages 44, 74), the Pigeon Posture (Page 107), the Modified Bow (Page 54), the Twist (Page 52), the Dancer's Posture (Page 58), the Cat Stretch (Pages 92-93), the Locust (Page 47).

WRESTLING AND JUDO

These sports harmoniously develop the muscles of the whole body, therefore, less supplemental training is required. However, both sports, but especially wrestling, insufficiently develop the pulmonary system (lungs). Inhalation and exhalations are not even, and often pressure occurs on the pulmonary system. The air in the gym or indoor sports environment is dusty, mats may not be clean, etc. These can also have negative effects on the athlete.

For wrestlers and judo athletes, the suggested exercises are:

- Raja Yoga exercises for controlling the mental and emotional states, and for developing concentration.
- YRE for speeding up the recovery process after hard training and competition (Page 126).
- Yoga breathing exercises: Abdominal and rhythmic yoga breathing with focus on inhalation and exhalation (Pages 137-138).
- Incorporate "Sitting still steadily" and concentration on the breathing, and one-two yoga asanas into your regular warm-up routine for both practicing concentration and for warm-up.
- Practicing autogenic training for withstanding the rigors of the intensive training (see Chapter 14).
- The Cobra (Pages 44, 74), the Bow (Page 68), the Locust (Page 47), the Twist (Page 52), the Pigeon Posture (Page 107). the Modified Camel Posture (Page 113), the Triangle (Pages 89-90), Seated Forward Bend (Page 69).

WEIGHTLIFTING (OLYMPIC)

This sport does not sufficiently develop the pulmonary system. The vital lung capacity of weight lifters is relatively low due to the pressure which develops on the pulmonary system during weightlifting. Weightlifters also experience dilation of capillarries and fallen arches. Yoga can help combat these problems.

For weightlifters, the suggested exercises are:

- Raja Yoga exercises for controlling the mental and emotional states and for developing concentration.

- YRE for speeding up the recovery process after hard training and competition (Page 126).

- Yoga breathing exercises: Abdominal breathing, rhythmic yoga breathing (Pages 137-138).

- Incorporate "sitting still steadily" and concentration on the breathing and one or two yoga asanas into your regular warm-up routine for both practicing concentration and for warm-up.

- Practicing autogenic training for withstanding the rigors of the intensive training (training load) (see Chapter 14).

- Abdominal life (Uddijana Bandha) and Nauli for decreasing the pressure in the stomach cavity (Page 81-83).

- Asanas in reverse position to prevent dilation of capillaries: The Shoulderstand, the Half Shoulderstand, (Pages 43, 67), the Headstand (Page 72).

- Sitting asanas and specific exercises to strengthen the muscles of the feet: the Resting Posture (Page 64), Half Lotus (Page 61), the Frog (Page 56), the Knee Bending Posture (Page 129), the Tiptoe Posture (Page 88).

- To stretch the muscles of back, legs, chest and stomach: Modified Sitting Forward Bend (Page 50), the Lunge (Page 106), the Cobra (Page 74), the Bow (Page 68), the Plough (Page 71), the Twist (Page 52). the Triangle (Pages 89-90). the Leg Stretch (Page 103), the Pigeon Posture (Page 107).

TEAM SPORTS

Team handball, basketball, volleyball, and football require less supplemental training and compensation exercises because of the positive effects these sports have on the development of the body.

For these athletes, the suggested exercises are:

- Raja Yoga exercises for controlling the mental and emotional states and for developing concentration.
- YRE for speeding up the recovery process after hard training and competition (Page 126).
- Yoga breathing exercises: Abdominal and rhythmic yoga breathing, the Double "R" Breath (Pages 137–138).
- Incorporate one or two yoga asanas and "Complete Yoga Breathing When Walking" (Page 137) into your regular warm-up routine for both practicing concentration and for warm-up.
- Practicing autogenic training for withstanding the rigors of the intensive hard training (see Chapters 14 and 15).
- Asanas affecting the spine to prevent back pain (Page 126).

SOCCER

This sport requires supplemental training. Since soccer is played predominantly by using the lower half of the body, those engaged in this sport need asanas which strengthen the upper body and the shoulders, especially for young players and asanas which affect the spine.

The suggested exercises for soccer players are:

- The Body Straight postures (Pages 99-105), the Crow (Page 86), the Side Crow (Page 87), the Cobra (Page 74), the Locust (Page 47), the Yoga Sit-up (Pages 110-111), the Modified Bow (Page 54), the Twisting Position (Page 51), the Twist (Page 52), the Triangle (Pages 89-90), the Bow (Page 68), the Plough (Page 71).

- YRE for speeding up the process of recovery after hard training and competition (Page 126).

- Yoga breathing exercises: Abdominal and rhythmic breathing, the double "R" breath, yoga breathing when walking (Pages 137-138).

- Incorporate one or two yoga asanas and the complete yoga breathing when walking into your regular warm-up routine for both practicing concentration and for warm-up.

- Raja Yoga exercises for controlling the mental and emotional states and for developing concentration.

- Asanas in sitting position for prevention of the development of deformation in the legs (legs in the shape of an "O").

TENNIS, RACQUET SPORTS

These sports belong in the one-sided sports category. Heavy use of the racquet arm can cause muscle dysbalance. Therefore, complex yoga training is recommended as supplemental and compensational training. These athletes need to focus on asanas that strengthen the lower back, and improve the flexibility of the shoulder and knee joints.

The suggested exercises are:

- Complete yoga training as supplemental and compensational training (Page 136).
- The Triangle (Pages 89-90), the Cobra (Pages 44, 74), the Locust (Page 47), the Modified Bow (Page 54), the Shoulder Stretch (Page 62), the Twisting Position (Page 51).
- Yoga breathing exercises: Abdominal breathing and rhythmic yoga breathing, the double "R" breathing, yoga breathing when walking (Page 137-138).
- YRE for speeding up the recovery process after hard training and competition (Page 126).
- Raja Yoga exercises for controlling the mental and emotional states and for developing concentration.
- Practicing autogenic training individually tailored for your specific needs (Chapter 14).

TRACK AND FIELD

Different events of track and field require different supplemental exercises. Decathlon athletes require less supplemental training.

WALKING, RUNNING

Simple cyclical movements like walking or running are "one-sided" from aspects of harmonious development. Therefore, complex yoga training as supplemental exercises is recommended.

In a race, one of the most important factors is synchronization of breathing phases with movement and optimum tempo. Systematic practice of breathing exercises helps the athlete to analyze his/her individual rhythm and feeling, experience the connection of movement with breathing, coordinate breathing with movement, and search for the optimum effect.

During running, the organs of the stomach are pulled down, which lowers the diaphragm, which, in turn, enhances inhalation. The position of the diaphragm is more favorable to inhalation than exhalation during running. More strength of the abdominal muscles is required for sufficient exhalation during running than during resting. The effect of this pulling down of the organs of the stomach cavity facilitating inhalation is felt during the landing or take-off phase of running. The effects on exhalation are felt during the flying phase.

The suggested exercises are:

- Asanas with reverse position, and which affect the spine for the prevention of pain in the lower back. Battery of yoga asanas for both rehabilitating the lower back, and prevention of pain and injury (Page 126), the Half Shoulderstand (Page 43), the Shoulderstand (Page 67), the Headstand (Page 72).

- Asanas which stretch the muscles of the thigh, calf and ankle: the Leg Stretch (Page 108), the Head to Knee Posture (Page 94), the Dancer's Posture (Page 58), the Seated Forward Bend (Page 69), the Modified Camel Posture (Page 113), the Lunge (Page 106).

- Yoga breathing exercises: Abdominal and rhythmic yoga breathing, yoga breathing when walking (Pages 137-138).

- YRE for speeding up the recovery process after hard training and competition (Page 126).

- Practicing autogenic training for withstanding the rigors of the intensive training (see Chapter 15).

- Raja Yoga exercises for controlling the mental and emotional states.

JUMPING EVENTS (LONG JUMP, HIGH JUMP, TRIPLE JUMP), THROWING EVENTS (SHOT PUT, JAVELIN, DISCUS)

In general, jumping and throwing events do not require involvement of the whole body. Therefore, it is necessary to practice supplemental exercises. In both jumping and throwing events, balance has a significant role. Sensations felt from the muscles and ligaments contribute greatly to the athletes sense of balance, therefore, yoga balance postures are recommended. By practicing these postures, a double effect is achieved—exercise of the whole body, and an increase sense of balance. These two effects facilitate improvement of sports performance.

Suggested exercises for throwing events:

- YRE for speeding up the recovery process (Page 126).

- Yoga breathing exercises: abdominal breathing, complete yoga breath (Pages 137-138).

- The Cobra (Page 74), The Bow (Page 68), the Triangle (89-90), Modified Sitting Forward Bend (Page 50), the Plough (Page 71), the Twist (Page 52), Abdominal Lift (Page 81), the Nauli (Page 82-83).

- Raja Yoga exercises for control of emotions, AT, TM.

Suggested exercises for jumping events:
- YRE for speeding up the recovery process (Page 126).

- Yoga breathing exercises: abdominal breathing, complete yoga breath (Pages 137-138).

- Asanas which affect the spine and strengthen the lower back: The Cobra (Page 74), The Bow (Page 68), the Triangle (89-90), the Twist (Page 52), the Locust (Page 47), the Cat Stretch (Pages 92-93).

- Transcendental Meditation, Autogenic Training.

7 ━━━━━

CLASSIFYING ASANAS

From the aspect of sport preparation, Hatha Yoga Asanas can be classified based on their effects. The following general categories of Asanas exist, i.e., Asanas which:

- support the normalization of body functions and stimulate and mobilize the different organs and glands (YSE);
- normalize and regenerate the functions of psychosomatic centers (plexuses) (YSE);
- increase the level of activation (YSE);
- deactivate and decrease the level of activation (calming) (YSE);
- compensate the muscle dysbalance that results from one sided loading (YCE);
- speed-up the process of regeneration (YRE);
- develop flexibility, elasticity, strength and endurance, etc. (YSE, YCE).

ASANAS THAT ACTIVATE AND DEACTIVATE

Examples of asanas and techniques which activate, or mobilize and stimulate, and tone the body. In general, rapid, strong breath (inhalation), open eyes, and leaning the trunk backward all have an activating effect.

Specific Activating Asanas:

- The Cobra (Page 74)
- The Locust (Page 47)
- The Bow (Page 68)
- The Half Shoulderstand (Page 43)
- The Modified Camel (Page 113)
- The Twist (Page 52)
- The Scale (Page 77)
- The Abdominal Lift (Page 81)
- Salutation to the Sun (Page 130-131)
- Kapalabhath Breathing Exercise

Examples of techniques which deactivate the body and have a relaxing calming effect.

In general, deep, slow, long exhalation, closed eyes and leaning the trunk forward all have a calming effect.

Specific Deactivating Asanas:

- The Modified Standing Forward Bend (Page 40)
- The Seated Forward Bend (Page 69)
- The Plough (Page 71)
- The Fish (Page 78)
- The Relaxation Posture (Page 84)
- Complete Yoga Breath (Page 26)
- Alternate Nostril Breath (Page 28)

BATTERY OF ASANAS FOR ACTIVATION (STIMULATION)

- The Cobra (Page 74)
- The Locust (Page 47)
- The Bow (Page 68)

BATTERY OF ASANAS FOR DEACTIVATION (CALMING)

- The Half Shoulderstand (Page 43)
- The Plough (Page 71)
- The Fish (Page 78)

In competition when athletes want to decrease their level of activation (high arousal level) and get into a deep, relaxed state, they should do it at the right time. The best time is 5-6 minutes after finishing their physical warm-up.

They can either use autogenic training (see chapter of autogenic training) or they can use the previously discussed deactivation techniques. This deep relaxation should always be followed by a series of short reactivation exercises in order to once again reach an optimal level of activation (in order to be once again prepared for competing). Both autogenic activation exercises and the above mentioned breathing exercises are suitable.

If the competition has longer breaks (e.g. repeated heats, starts, qualification bouts, etc.) the athletes should rest and restore their strength and energy. They can do this either using autogenic training specifically for the recovery of strength, or employing the YRE techniques found in Chapter 6.

Sometimes it is necessary to go through another warm-up (if there is a long pause in the competition). Athletes should plan these additional warm-ups so that they reach the desired state of preparedness without wasting too much energy. Each warm-up battery should be individual and sport specific.

8 ▬▬▬

GUIDELINES, PRINCIPLES FOR DESIGNING YOUR PROGRAM

It is necessary to gain the ability to create your own batteries based on your concrete needs and goals. Selection of asana should be sport and individual specific. You can use the batteries of asanas presented in this book. You will find it very beneficial as many did.

Following are some of the main guidelines you should keep in mind.

- Consider your experience in yoga. Are you a beginner or advanced student?
- Set your goals. What is the primary goal you want to achieve with the battery of asanas? (e.g., speeding up the process of regeneration, calming, relaxing your body-mind, compensating muscle dysbalance or increasing your flexibility, elasticity, etc.) Remember with yoga you can simultaneously achieve more than one goal.
- A general yoga routine should start with a sitting posture suitable for meditation. Starting the routine with a short meditation will lead to heightened concentration during the entire practice.
- Try to start your regular sport training with short meditation as part of your regular warm-up. This meditation will be a transition to the concentration required for your training or competition. It will help with calm analysis of the situation or problem at hand or even competition. It will enhance clear thinking and eliminate anxiety and stress.

A GENERAL YOGA ROUTINE

- Start with asanas which stretch and relax the limbs and strengthen the muscles, ligaments and joints.

- The routines should include asanas for exercising the spine (different bends: forward, backward, side, rotation executed in standing, sitting or lying positions).

- The routine should further include at least one asana in a reverse position (shoulder stand, head stand, etc.) and an Asana which compresses the stomach cavity (abdominal lift, etc.).

- Autogenic self-suggestive verbal phrases and mental imagery should be used also to affect the body.

- When you execute a yoga asana, use autogenic verbal phrases to increase the biological effect of the asana, the function of your muscles and body.

- Repeat the autogenic verbal phrases in your mind very slowly in a monotone way without any accent. After each verbal phrase pause, then repeat the phrase more times.

- Yoga asanas are 80 percent mental and 20 percent physical. Practicing yoga asanas is like meditation.

- After these asanas, the body and the mind are prepared for breathing exercises and for meditation, which will bring the mind more under control.

- Relaxation as a transition to normal daily activity should terminate each yoga program. However, the relaxation must be terminated with short activation exercises (re-activation).

- Usually, the routine starts with one of the easier asanas.

- In the morning, asanas with accentuating and stimulating effects should be selected, with less demand on flexibility of joints. In the evening due to overall "warm-up" of the body and general fatigue, asanas with high demand on flexibility of joints are selected.

- When practicing asanas with a forward bend (flexion), it is necessary to compensate with backward bending asanas (extension).

- A general rule of breathing is that you exhale when you contract your belly and the front side of your body, and inhale when you contract your back (that is, if you bend your trunk forward you exhale; when you lean your trunk back you inhale) when maintaining the posture breath regularly.

- Rotation to one side should be practiced with rotation of the opposite side.

- Do not practice sooner than one and a half to two hours after eating.

- After hard training, use only YRE. Only later schedule a bigger yoga routine at home.

(More suggestions on developing your own yoga routine are found in Chapter 16)

PART IV

TRAINING THE
TOTAL ATHLETE

9

SELF-STUDY: LEARNING CONTROL THROUGH LEARNING YOURSELF

Self-control starts with self-study. In order to regulate your mind and mental state, you must first understand it. The way to do this is through self-study, self-observation, and education.

Self-education is a life-long process. You can use it to develop you physical, mental, intellectual, and moral qualities. The key to getting to know yourself is a willingness to look thoroughly into yourself, take responsibility for your mental state, and be open to changing it. This requires courage and commitment. Only you can control yourself. No one else can do it for you. This takes work! But the rewards can be great. First, you will gain more control over your performance; second, you will be able to take more control over other responsibilities in your life, such as school, work, or family life.

There are many ways to educate or study yourself. You should try as many as possible.

Yoga is an excellent means for self-observation, self-study, and self-education. The static nature of yoga asanas and the way in which yoga is practiced—the focused concentration and introspection—give excellent opportunity for self-observation, noticing and experiencing different bodily functions, sensations, muscle tensions, turning the mind inward during meditation we learn the nature of self. When you assume a yoga posture, you tune out the outside world and turn your focus inward. This allows you to heighten your proprioceptive sense. In short, yoga is biofeedback with the modern electronic equipment.

READING BIOGRAPHIES

Reading the biographies and autobiographies of famous athletes can be very helpful. Books provide you with role models for your own achievements in sport. You can also learn through reading that many top athletes systematically record in detail their observations, feelings and actions. (Biographies of high achievers in art, science and yoga masters are also useful.)

THE RIGHT ATTITUDE

An important part of self-analysis is identifying your attitude toward your sport. Why are you involved? What do you get out of your participation? How you look at your sport in relation to the rest of your life can have a major impact on your performance.

In my experience, those athletes who place an undue amount of importance on their results suffer. On the other hand, those who achieve stable, constant performances look at their sport as an important, but not the only, part of their life. They enjoy the fight, the mental game, the moment-to-moment experience. Regardless of the athlete's level, the reward—the enjoyment, happiness, and satisfaction—comes from the challenge and ongoing encounter with the sport and from the long term progress, improvement, and development. The experience and development rather than winning or losing is what motivates top athletes.

SETTING GOALS

Learning more about yourself will enable you to set realistic goals. Conversely, setting goals will help you gain additional insight. Goal setting can be formal or informal—whatever works for you. But don't let it take the fun out of your sport.

Set goals with your coach. He or she has the best handle on your present technical and tactical qualities and what goals would be challenging and realistic for you. Working with your coach will help ensure that you avoid setting goals that are incompatible with your ability. You should set more than just performance goals. Set objectives for technical, tactical, physical, mental, and behavioral development as well as goals related to diet and sleep. If you do not have a coach, analyze your training diary, your strengths, and weaknesses. Based on this analysis you can set your own realistic goals. You can also consult with fellow athletes.

The next step is determining a path that will lead you toward attainment of the goals. Effectively organize your daily regimen. Plan a one-year training program that includes monthly, weekly, and daily objectives. If you systematically keep the designed daily regimen, you will develop a positive habit of discipline and self-control and the ability to effectively organize your time. Even if you cannot keep precisely to the plan, you will learn more about yourself. This is information that you would have never obtained if you had not set goals in the first place. In any case, systematic evaluation of your activities increases your responsibility for fulfilling these objectives, provides you with feedback for revising your plan, and allows you to recognize your accomplishments.

A TRAINING DIARY

Another extremely useful tool in self-study is a training diary. In the diary you should record everything—your goals, your training load, the time, the quantity of work, and the intensity of your training. Also record the way that you react to certain situations, your reactions to stress, the physical, mental, and emotional changes that you undergo during training or competition, etc. Keep notes about your performances—your thoughts, observations, and feelings. You should analyze your actions, thoughts, and the objective facts about your performances, so that you get in the habit of self-study and self-education.

Many athletes I have worked with have found that they were unaware of what was blocking their progress. However, they recognized that the training diary was a helpful tool. For example, one athlete learned that he had muscle tension that he had not been aware of at all. He said, "If I had not kept a log, I would have never known that I was tense. Awareness has helped me to relax. Now, because I am tuned in, I notice when I am tight, and can say, 'Just take a deep breath and let it go.'"

As you observe and record these things in your training diary, you should analyze how you are doing. Are you training at the right level of intensity? Objectively speaking, how successful are you right now? Evaluate your weaknesses in the physical, mental, technical, and tactical areas. What are the obstacles that interfere with your greater achievement in sport?

RECORD YOUR DAILY ROUTINE IN YOUR TRAINING DIARY

It is also important to effectively organize your time and your daily routine. If you regularly keep to the routine that you have designed for yourself, you will develop positive habits of discipline, self-control, and the ability to effectively organize your time.

Set daily goals and give yourself voluntary tasks, in writing, to do in a certain time period. Verbally and in writing, evaluate your training sessions, your performances, and your actions. Regularly evaluating your activity increases your sense of responsibility for fulfilling your daily goals and tasks. If you do this, you will learn to give a daily account to yourself of how you are doing. It is like giving a "receipt" to yourself and to your coach about your activities and development.

Putting your self-analysis into writing will help you understand the causes of your failures and successes. Through it, you will develop better self-knowledge and self-awareness. You'll learn to better understand yourself, and you'll discover the source of your errors. You can also learn to solve your inner conflicts.

Sometimes, simply recording your difficulties in your training diary may provide some relief. Trying to look at difficulties more objectively (in writing), gives you a more systematic way of finding the reason(s) for your problems.

It is a good idea to record and utilize the opinions, notes, and observations of others about your performance. This type of self-study involves learning from your critics. Observations from teammates, coaches, opponents, friends, etc. can be very useful. The occasional off-hand comment from other people is usually more valuable than answers to your direct questions. For instance, the comment that "He always does the same action," may say a lot to you.

OBSERVING YOUR BODY, LEARNING YOUR BODY LANGUAGE

To have consistency in your performance, it is important to develop control over your physical, mental, and emotional states. The first step in developing self-control is getting to know yourself—the nature of your mind, your body language, and the mind-body relationship.

Yoga is one of the best means for achieving this important goal. When you assume a yoga posture, you tune out the outside world and turn your focus inward. This allows you to heighten your proprioceptive senses (perceptual awareness of your internal physical environment). These techniques are discussed in detail in Chapter 2.

In addition to yoga postures, Kundalini Yoga exercises are useful for improving body awareness. Kundalini Yoga deals with maintaining the functions of physical organs and bringing into awareness the organs' feeling due to their function. The task is to focus the attention on different body areas or organs and on the feelings generated in these areas in different life situations. Concentrative analysis, described in Chapter 12, is a modification of such Kundalini exercises. The main emphasis of these exercises is to focus attention on a particular area of the body and to concentrate on and observe the sensations that occur during different situations.

Biofeedback provides another technique for developing body awareness. This is done through the use of scientific monitoring devices that provide specific information (such as skin temperature or heart rate).

An important step in self-study is self-observation. You may start by observing these things about yourself:

General Bodily Sensations: Start observing your body functions—your breathing, your heartbeat, and the tension in your muscles. You can learn to distinguish feelings of tension, relaxation, warmth, and other sensations very accurately.

Specific Bodily Sensations: First, observe your breathing pattern, your heartbeat, and your muscle tension in a resting state. Observe any other sensations. Then begin to observe your physical sensations in other situation: when taking an important exam or interview; before an important competition; when you are relaxed and happy; when you are angry or unhappy.

MISPLACED ACTIVITY AND NERVOUS HABITS

Very often you will experience misplaced tension—tension where you don't expect it. You may tense those muscles in your sport which should be relaxed. For example, you may get tension in your shoulder when you serve a tennis ball. This misplaced tension is very important for you to know about. Misplaced tension and effort can lead to poor technique, fatigue, pain, or even injury. Observing when and with what movements you misplace effort or tension, can be extremely helpful to you.

Observe whether you have nervous habits which burn up your energy: tapping your feet; restless pacing; gum chewing. Do you have useless actions? Observe yourself during the day, and notice when you have misplaced tension in your body; identify activities which burn up your physical and emotional energy.

OBSERVING HOW YOUR BODY RESPONDS TO STRESS

Each of us responds to stress in a different way. Observe yourself before an important competition, and ask yourself some questions. Did your heart rate increase? Did you feel tension in your muscles? In which muscle groups did you feel the tension? Did your palms sweat? Did you feel cold sweat? Did you have a nervous stomach? How long does it take for the systems to return to your normal (pre-event) level?

The objective of this is not to make you worry. Observation helps you discover which of your systems respond to stress. Observing and identifying your response, is the first step in regulating your body and mind. You should also observe and identify the thoughts, images, and feelings that you associate with your body's responses. Think about it. How can you use your breathing rate, your heart rate, muscle tension ,and/or misplaced effort to tell you about your mental state? In this manual you will learn how to calm yourself, relax yourself, get rid of unnecessary tension, etc. But first you must become aware of what is happening in your body and how you respond to stress.

Observe your sensations, the mentioned respond to stress when you achieve your best results, when you had your best performance, bout, or game. Then, observe when you performed your worst. What was the difference in sensations?

Similarly, observe your thoughts, images, self-talk when you did your best and worst. What was the difference?

UNDERSTANDING YOUR SUBCONSCIOUS MIND

Through introspection you can learn more about your subconscious mind. We all have recurring patterns of thinking. Understanding them can help us to break free from the thoughts that hold us back. The following Raja Yoga exercise will help you to learn more about your thought patterns.

EXERCISE

- In a quiet place, assume a comfortable sitting position. It can be a simple cross-legged position or sitting on a chair. Keep your spine, neck, and head aligned. Rest your hands on your knees, with the thumb of each hand lightly touching the tip of the forefinger. Close your eyes, but do not squeeze them shut.

- Now allow all your muscles to relax. Be aware of your body sitting still—motionless and relaxed.

- Become aware of your breathing. Do not change or manipulate it—just be aware of its natural rhythm.

- Practice concentration in this posture for 3-4 minutes. Choose a spot on the wall or an object you like, such as a flower or a vase, and gaze at it. Or just concentrate on your breathing without manipulating it. Just feel your belly moving in and out or focus on the space under your nostrils where the air enters and leaves your body as you breath in and out. Do not force concentration. Let it happen.

- If you find (and you will) that your mind is wandering, simply be aware of the thought. Do not fight or suppress it. Just come back gently to your breathing or to your object of concentration.

- Your thoughts will flow like a stream of water—one after the other. Observe them in a detached manner. You may notice that individual thoughts will come and go, and do not last long.

- Take note of whether your thoughts are about the past—particularly unsuccessful performances—or future, and what emotions are attached to them, such as anger or worry.

- Take note of thoughts that bring you feelings of fear and worry.

- Notice how some thoughts come back.

- Notice how feelings and moods are associated with certain thoughts.

- Notice that bodily sensations and physical discomfort (for example, tension and pain in the shoulders, back, and ankles) can disturb your concentration as well.

- Use these bodily sensations as teaching tools in learning about yourself. By accepting physical discomfort as part of your experience in the moment, you can learn it is possible to relax and concentrate and to use it as a learning device. They can help you to develop your inner strength and your power of concentration.

- Notice that every time your mind moves, so does your body. If your mind is restless, your body will be as well (and vice versa).

You will notice that the stream of thoughts that enters your mind varies in nature. If you are in a high-stress state, such as before an important competition, your thoughts can be charged with anxiety and worry. Thoughts can also be less anxious in nature but powerful enough to draw your attention from the object of concentration.

From these exercises you can draw an important conclusion: becoming aware that thoughts come in and go out of your mind, and that these thoughts are not "you," will help you discover the nature of the mind, the constant thought processing, and also that you can choose to relate to or ignore particular thoughts. You will become more aware that what counts is not what you are thinking, but how you react to those thoughts. Learning to become more detached from your thoughts will allow you to become liberated from the "tyranny of thought" that many experience.

For example, a tennis player preparing to serve may have the thought that she may double fault. This thought can cause anxiety and turn into reality. On the other hand, if you let this negative thought pass by and supplement it with a positive one (for example: "hit the serve deep"), the positive tack will turn into reality.

SHARPENING VOLUNTARY ATTENTION SKILLS

Concentration and meditation are the steps that lead to self-control. A precondition of concentration is voluntary attention based on self-discipline. That means that you must be fully attuned to what you are doing. The following Kundalini Yoga exercises can help you to become more fully attuned by requiring that you pay full attention to what you are doing.

Many of us pay little attention to basic activities such as eating. Our attention is everywhere as we mechanically load our stomachs while watching television or reading. As a result, we don't experience the natural feeling of fullness, and find ourselves feeling stuffed later.

The following simple exercise can help you to be aware of what total attention means, as well as to improve your eating habits. Weight sensitive athletes in sports such as boxing, wrestling, and gymnastics find this particularly helpful.

EXERCISE ONE
- Take a food that you like—for example, an orange.
- Focus your attention on the orange. Observe it. Notice the color, the shape, and the size. Feel the texture. Notice the skin. Now peel the orange, noticing the texture. Put a section in your mouth and notice the taste and temperature.
- Chew it slowly, thoroughly, and carefully with full concentration. Notice the taste, temperature, and textures as you chew it. Notice the amount of salivation that occurs in your

mouth. Notice the process of swallowing consciously. Take another bite only after you finish swallowing completely.

A similar exercise involves observing the process of drinking. As you do this exercise think of the professional wine taster, paying attention to every detail of the experience.

EXERCISE TWO

- Take a small amount of water or tea into your mouth.
- First become aware of sensations (taste and temperature) in the mouth. Then swallow a small amount slowly.
- Observe how the water or tea moves down the throat. In the case of cold or warm liquid you might also feel the momentum of it entering the stomach.

When you first do this exercise, you may not observe very many specifics but over time, more and more details will come into your awareness.

The results of both exercises will be that when eating or drinking, the brain cortex's influence—that is, the mental image of appetite—will have less influence and the natural feeling of hunger or thirst will come into the foreground. As a result, the food or liquid intake will be more precisely regulated.

Another Kundalini technique (organ awareness) consists of observation of the feelings and sensations of the organs. The task is to focus the attention on various parts of the body during various routine events such as sexual function, digestion, eating, drinking, and so on. The idea is to observe what feelings you experience in related organs.

Learn to pay full attention to what you are doing. The Kundalini exercises mentioned above are very useful. You might discover that you use food for your emotional comfort, especially when you feel anxious, or that you take all your troubles with you when going to sleep, or that you do not pay full attention to what you are doing, or that you are not mentally where you are physically.

Try observing how easily your own awareness is carried away from the present moment by your thoughts. Notice how much of the time during the day you find yourself thinking about the past or about the future, instead of focusing on what you are doing now. As you will see in Chapter 15, athletes I interviewed were surprised at how much was going on in their minds during competition.

OBSERVING THE FUNCTION OF PERCEPTIONS AND COGNITION

A higher degree of self-observation comes with observing the functions of perception and cognition. Observe how you are concentrating on what you are doing. Is your mind wandering and distracted? Can you fully concentrate on the task or activity at hand, or does your concentration slip away? Do you have negative thoughts and self-talk during competition? What thoughts? When? Keep track of your thoughts and self-talk. Record them in your training diary.

Active self-observation of the emotional state can have an impact on how we feel. For example, it is impossible to be angry and at the same time to make self-observations. Self-observation "freezes" the effects of the emotions. When we start to observe ourselves, we simultaneously begin to control ourselves. For example, try to start self-observation in a moment of uncontrollable laughter and you will see how the intensity and spontaneity of the laugher will decrease.

Unfortunately, the effect of negative emotions such as fear and anxiety does not disappear with simple self-observation. On the contrary, these emotions have the ability to increase the severity of emotions. Here it is necessary to find and eliminate the reason for the emotions. Self-observation is a good start for this.

Each area of your life, especially your sport performance, is influenced by your emotions, thoughts, attitudes, and feelings. And you know that success in sports is greatly determined by how you are able to control your emotions.

AWARENESS OF THE DEGREE OF MUSCULAR TENSION — "KINESTHETIC TRAINING"

Another area of self-observation and self-study involves awareness of your muscular tension and physical "effort." It is very important for you to be in a "relaxed" state during competition. If you are tense, your movements will be stiff or awkward, and you will tire easily. However, athletic effort requires tension in the right muscles while you are performing. Training yourself to be aware of the degree of tension in your various muscle groups will help both your technique and your endurance. Training yourself in body awareness and muscular tension is called kinesthetic training.

Kinesthetic training means isometric contraction of a certain muscle group with varying degrees (effort) and then total relaxation of muscles.

In kinesthetic training you contract a particular muscle group for a few seconds, and then totally relax the area. The objective is to experience the changes as fully as possible. With practice, you should be able to develop a heightened awareness between the various degrees of tension and relaxation. This awareness of the difference between the two states and between the various degrees of muscle tension is referred to as kinesthetic differentiation. Concentration and de-concentration is based on similar principles as tension and relaxation, but on a mental rather than physical level.

Developing awareness between the tense muscle state and the relaxed muscle state is essential to learning and performing sports activities. When competing or learning a new movement, we all have experienced "trying too hard," or using too much conscious effort. This leads to tensing inappropriate muscle groups resulting in uncoordinated, stiff movements. Learning kinesthetic differentiation is the basis for developing the proper sense of how much effort to use in any particular situation.

Kinesthetic training is also important for learning and perfecting the techniques and skills of sport. Heightened kinesthetic awareness helps in:

- minimizing energy consumption
- coordinating movements
- relaxation and rejuvenation

For the following discussion you need to understand that there are three different types of muscle tension. First, tonic tension is the increased level of tension in muscles in the resting state due to stress and anxiety. Second, speed tension occurs especially in movements that are executed at maximum speed. Under these conditions muscles are not able to relax completely. The change from muscle tension to relaxation occurs more slowly than the change from relaxation to muscle tension. As a result, in a certain phase of the movement the muscles doing the work will be tense as will the antagonistic muscles. This conflict reduces the speed of the movement. Third, coordination tension occurs when an individual is learning new movements or skills; unwanted tension results from the uncertainty of movement.

The following exercises will help you develop kinesthetic differentiation.

EXERCISE ONE

- Sit or lie in a comfortable position. Close your eyes.

- Spread the fingers of one hand as far apart as possible while arching the wrist backward. Take a deep breath and keep your forearm, hand, and fingers tense for 4 to 5 seconds. Observe and feel the tension in your fingers and hand. Now exhale slowly and let the tension go. Relax the muscles in your fingers, hand, and forearm. Observe how different this feeling is from the feeling of tension.

- Make a fist with your dominant hand. Tighten the muscles while taking a deep breath. Hold this position for 4 to 5 seconds. Become fully aware of the sensation of your hand tightening. Now exhale slowly and relax the muscles in your hand. Let it go. Now repeat this exercise using each of the major muscle groups in the body.

- Repeat the previous two exercises (with the same muscle groups) with one variation: use a lesser degree of tension in the tense phase of the action. However, you should still concentrate on the difference between the state of tension and the state of relaxation. Repeat the exercise several more times, each time using a lesser degree of tension.

- Now repeat the same exercise using various muscle groups that are most often tensed in response to stress in your sport. Be specific and concentrate on problem areas that you have.

The following are examples of what to do to help when too much tension develops in a particular muscle group, for example shoulder tension when cutting or thrusting in fencing:

- Shoulders: Raise your shoulders to your ears, holding the tension, then relax. Repeat while applying less and less degree of tension.
- Neck: Tilt your head backward and tense the muscles in your neck. Hold the tension and then relax. Now tilt your head forward, until your chin touches your chest, while tensing the muscles in the back of your neck. Hold the tension and then relax. Repeat, applying less tension each time.
- Face: Although the facial muscles are not directly involved in many sports, stress and anxiety often manifest themselves through facial tension. Relaxing your facial muscles helps to relieve the tension. Begin this exercise by frowning. Hold the muscles in your face tense and then relax. Now tighten or squeeze the muscles around your eyes and forehead. Hold this position and relax. Repeat, applying less tension each time. Then tighten the muscles around your mouth and jaw by clenching the jaw then relaxing it.

You and your coach together should design a concrete set of exercises that work with specific muscle groups important to your sport. If you do not have a coach, study what muscle groups are involved in your sport, which have the main role, which muscles should be relaxed. Also, analyze your training diary, which activities cause misplaced tension and which muscles you tighten. They should also be individualized, since every athlete manifests tension in a different way. This relaxation exercise is most effective in counteracting the effects of tonic tension.

EXERCISE TWO

Another type of exercise that can increase kinesthetic differentiation is the progressive release of tension in a particular muscle group. The sense of relaxation can be enhanced by linking the sensation of relaxation with the physical movement of dropping a particular limb or muscle group as a result of gravity. Tying the movement to the feeling of relaxation helps to solidify the relationship. In this type of exercise, the muscle group is contracted and then slowly released in increments. As the muscle slowly relaxes, the sensation of tension is transformed into a feeling of heaviness; as the muscles relax, they are affected by the force of gravity. The following is an example of such an exercise.

- Stand with the feet shoulder-width apart and the arms hanging loosely beside the body.
- Now bend forward until the trunk is parallel to the ground. As you are bending forward, raise the arms to the side until they are also parallel to the ground.
- Tense the muscles in your arms and shoulders and make fists.
- Relax the muscles in your arms, shoulders, and hands completely. Feel how your muscles gradually release the tension.
- Let gravity pull your arms down until they are totally loose. As gravity pulls your arms, feel the release of the tension. Notice that gravity helps you relax.

You can construct similar exercises for the legs.

EXERCISE THREE

In the next step you can practice exercises in which the change in tension goes from tension to relaxation in a slow and gradual manner. The Cobra is an excellent example. An example is as follows:

- Lie on your stomach with your forehead on the floor and your arms at your sides.

- Inhale and slowly raise your head, stretching forward and upward. At the same time also raise your shoulders. Hold this position for 3 to 4 seconds.
- Now place your hands on the floor shoulder-width apart and underneath your shoulders. Your arms should be bent.
- From this position, continue to raise your chest and head, using your arms to support you. Do not go so far as to raise your stomach off the floor.
- Breath evenly and maintain this position for a few seconds.
- Now exhale slowly and lower your upper body, slowly releasing the tension.
- When your head reaches the floor, relax and hold this position for a few moments.
- Now repeat this sequence three separate times. At the end, bring your arms down to your sides and next to your body, and relax completely.

EXERCISE FOUR

Once you have learned the exercises for relaxing muscles gradually, practice an exercise in which you suddenly change the state of your muscle from tense to relaxed. The Locust will accomplish this for you:

- First lie on your stomach. Rest your chin on the floor and place your hands, which are in fists, near your sides.
- Now inhale, push your fists down onto the floor, and raise both legs as high as possible. Breathe evenly and hold this position for 5 seconds.
- Exhale and lower your legs, allowing gravity to do the work. Repeat this exercise three times.

You can also create your own sport-specific kinesthetic exercises. For example, in fencing, a common problem is excess tension in the shoulder and arm muscles that occurs when the fencer is thrusting. The fencer can practice eliminating this problem by doing the following exercise.

The fencer thrusts and hits either a dummy target or the coach. After contact is made the student consciously unlocks his or her elbow, helping to release the tension in the shoulder and arm area. Concentrating on unlocking the elbow helps to relax the arm and shoulder area. The athlete should concentrate on the sensations as they are occurring.

The following exercises are example of how to increase awareness of sudden change from tension to relaxation:

- While jumping rope, pay special attention to the relaxation in your feet and your legs that occurs immediately after you jump.
- When dribbling a basketball, try to relax your wrist and arm after each contact with the ball.
- When throwing the medicine ball, concentrate your attention on relaxing the muscles of your hand and arm immediately after each throw.

OTHER METHODS FOR DEVELOPING KINESTHETIC AWARENESS

You can also heighten your kinesthetic awareness by any of the following methods:

- Practice some actions of your sport blindfolded — for example, dribbling a basketball.
- Practice your sport using equipment that is slightly different in either size or weight in order to gain awareness of the differences. (For example, use a heavier racquet in tennis or a smaller ball in soccer.)
- Simply review your movements in your mind, especially when movements have been incorrectly executed. Try and discern exactly what happened. Was there too much tension in your arm, shoulder, etc.?

- Describe to your coach how well you think you executed a movement and what you think you did right and wrong. Now compare your perception with your coach's. You can learn from both the commonalties and the discrepancies.
- Work with the coach in actually trying to change your technique.
- Explore yoga exercises (see Chapter 2) and biofeedback.
- Observe and record subjective feelings and images after executing particular moves.
- Periodically review the correct techniques of your sport.

Another invaluable tool in the process of self-study is biofeedback. Biofeedback is "hi-tech" yoga, or a "hi-tech" way of doing self-observation. Biofeedback sensors can tell you about tiny changes in your level of relaxation, tension, arousal, or excitement.

Biofeedback is a convincing tool for helping you understand that passive attention, attending to the process without striving or trying to "let it happen," is the technique to control your autonomic, or involuntary, functions. Through biofeedback, you will more easily understand the power of image (intention).

The autogenic exercises below demonstrate the power of imaging (intention) to accomplish results (for example, to produce unconscious muscular activity, or to inhibit voluntary action) if you focus passively without strain or striving—if you let the process just happen. Practice the exercises one by one until you are successful at them. Concentrate passively, have a let-it-happen attitude.

Focus on the process of what you are doing and not on how well you are doing the exercise. Use your imagination—be like an actor seeing himself or herself performing a role.

THE PENDULUM EXERCISE

For this exercise, you will need a small, light object such as a ring or a small ball. Tie a thread or chain about six inches long to the object. Hold the thread or chain between your thumb and forefinger, with your elbow resting on a table or the arm of your chair. Then imagine (have the intention) that the pendulum is moving from right to left or back and forth. Notice how the image in your mind produces movement of the pendulum in the imagined direction. You can then change your image (intention) (while the pendulum is still swinging) of the pendulum moving the opposite way.

This exercise demonstrates how an intention or an idea or mental image innervates a certain muscle group. The idea or image in your mind generates impulses in the nervous system and produces unconscious muscular activity.

THE BALLOON EXERCISE

You can get a similar effect of involuntary (ideomotor) muscle movement in your arms. Extend your arms out straight in front of you at shoulder level. Close your eyes and imagine a heavy piece of iron tied to your right hand; then imagine a big balloon fixed to your left hand. Envision how this big balloon, filled with gas, is lifting your arm and how it is floating upward. Next, feel how the heavy iron is drawing your right arm down.

THE CLOSED-EYE EXERCISE

Sit or lie down in a comfortable position, close your eyes, and concentrate on relaxing your whole body. Next, with your eyes still closed, roll your eyeballs upward and "focus" on your forehead. Repeat to yourself for approximately 2 minutes, *"My eyes are closed."* While still repeating this phrase, tell yourself to open your eyes. You will find that you cannot.

This exercise demonstrates how a voluntary action can be inhibited by thinking of another, incompatible idea. Telling yourself that your eyes are closed blocks the neurological activity that is needed to open the eyes.

THE HEAVINESS EXERCISE

Sit or lie in a comfortable position. Place your dominant hand on your dominant thigh (for example, if you are right handed, put your right hand on your right thigh). Close your eyes and relax your body. Imagine a heavy weight attached to your arm pulling your arm down toward the ground. Also vividly imagine how the weight is pulling your body down, more and more, and how your hand and arm are sliding down. Now repeat to yourself, "*My arm is heavy, very heavy.*" Each time you repeat the word "heavy," imagine the heavy weight pulling your arm down. In this exercise, you are conditioning yourself to associate the sensation of heaviness with the word "heavy."

THE WARMTH EXERCISE

Assume a comfortable sitting position. Sit still. Relax. Place your hands on your lap, and hold an ordinary thermometer between the thumb and forefinger of your dominant hand. Close your eyes. Focus your attention on your breathing. Now have an intention to get your dominant hand warmer. Imagine touching a hot stove or resting on the beach under the sun, whatever image you prefer. Do not strive or strain, just focus on your breathing and hold your image. Let it happen. After a while, notice the thermometer. The temperature will be higher than before.

THE COLD EXERCISE

In the same position as above now have the intention of getting your hand, cold. Imagine that you are holding a snowball which freezes your hand. or use any other image you prefer. Each time you inhale notice and feel the cold air in your nostrils. After a few minutes, notice the thermometer. You will notice a decrease by a few degrees. (Try again for a few more minutes if you do not notice any change.)

THE HEARTBEAT EXERCISE

In the same position as above, imagine visualize that you are running after a train you desperately must catch, or imagine that you are running your last round to win the gold medal and your opponent is slightly ahead of you. Notice the increased pulse rate on the pulse meter attached to your index finger.

To Decrease Your Heart Rate: Induce the image of resting in your bedroom and taking a nap.

How powerful such images (intentions) can be was demonstrated by the famous Russian neurologist A.R. Luria. Luria reported the remarkable abilities of his famous subject who was able to change all kinds of involuntary functions. He could raise and lower the temperature of his hand by simply visualizing touching a warm stove with his hand or holding a piece of ice. He could change his heartbeat by imagining running after a train as it pulled out of a station or imagining lying in bed talking a nap. He could contract or dilate his pupils by imagining himself staring at the sun or sitting in he dark.

Through self-study you will learn the extreme importance of awareness. You will learn also, that awareness can be trained.

To control your muscle tension and emotions you must be aware of them first. What is outside of awareness you cannot control. It is the power of awareness you use when you decide to switch from involuntary (for example, irregular) breathing to voluntary (for example, deep, regular) breathing, or when you relax your shoulders when serving in tennis.

By using awareness you can correct the errors and distortions in your performance.

Every intention is a trigger for transformation—for change. As your awareness switches and you intend to do something, your nervous system responds to achieving this goal.

By increasing your awareness, bringing into a new focus, you can alter your emotional state, your performance. As Deepak Chopra pointed out in his 1993 book *Ageless Body, Timeless Mind*, new awareness produces new biochemistry.

Your internal programming is unconscious, so you do not realize the tremendous effect of awareness on staying relaxed, being alert, confident, calm in almost all aspects of your life.

You can consciously use awareness to your benefit.

10

SELF-CONTROL THROUGH YOGA: RAJA YOGA AND MENTAL CONTROL

I consider Raja Yoga techniques the most perfect means for gaining self-control, and I incorporate these techniques into the mental training program for my students.

The ultimate goal of Raja Yoga is to clear the mind from thoughts, images, and desires. This is achieved through eight steps described in the first written synthesis of yoga—the *Pantanjai's Yoga Sutras*: *yamas*, or restraints; *niyamas*, or observances; *asanas*, or postures, *pranayama*, regulation of breath; *pratyhara,* or drawing the senses inward; *dharana*, or concentration, *dhyana*, or meditation; *samadhi*, or superconsciousness. I adapted some of these steps into the following series of exercises: (See Chapter 2 also.)

1. Body awareness—control through Yoga postures
2. Breath awareness—control—through Yoga breathing exercises
3. Voluntary attention focus—control through self-discipline
4. Concentration

These exercises will lead to more control over the mind and body (see Table 5 on page 5). Practiced individually, each element will be helpful, but together the program is even more powerful. Each step enhances the other. Table 6 (page 6) shows the inner relationship among the steps and exercises. Body control facilitates breath control, and conversely, breath control facilitates body control. Similarly, body and breath control facilitate voluntary attention focus, and attention focus leads to the development of concentration. Also, practicing each of the four steps leads to improvement of each of the other skills.

Body Awareness (Control) Through Yoga Postures

The following examples will show you how I guide my students in developing body control through yoga postures. In the previous chapters, I already discussed how to execute a yoga posture, and how to enhance body control through asanas. My athletes start their training and competition with sitting still steadily and concentrating on their breathing. Athletes have told me that simply "sitting still steadily" or practicing breath awareness can be of immediate help in controlling the mental state. This is the first exercise that my students use to start each practice or competition.

Exercise

Assume a comfortable sitting position in a quiet place. It can be a simple cross-legged position. Keep your spine, neck, and head aligned with each other. Rest your hands on your knees, with the thumb of each hand lightly touching the tip of the forefinger. Gently close your eyes, but do not squeeze them shut.

If the cross-legged position is uncomfortable, sit on a wooden chair. Make sure your trunk, neck, and head are erect, and firmly place your feet flat on the floor. Whatever position you take, it must include a straight back, aligned with the neck and head in a comfortable position, and easy breathing.

Sit still steadily. Do not move. The mind and body are one. When your body moves, your mind moves, and vice versa. Be aware of your body sitting still, motionless, and relaxed. Make sure that your sitting position is still comfortable, relaxed, and steady.

Now relax all your muscles. Visualize and allow all your muscles to relax, to become soft, loose. Start from the top of your head, and visualize and relax the muscles of your forehead, the muscles around your eyes, mouth, the facial muscles, and the muscles of your neck, shoulders, arms, and hands. Go progressively through each part of your body as you learned in kinestethic training. Relax the muscles of your chest, back, the abdominal muscles, and the muscles around your hips and pelvis the muscles of your thighs, knees, calves, and feet. Scan your body and if you notice any tension, just flow relaxation to this area as you quietly exhale. You can repeat this procedure one more time.

Take more deep, comfortable breaths and attune to your body. Sit still quietly—this steady, relaxed position will still and calm your body. You will become aware of different physical sensations like twitches or heaviness.

Sitting still will help you develop breath awareness and concentration, control thoughts and emotions, and eliminate external distractions. Later, you will also use this position to practice yoga breathing, concentration, and meditation.

Sitting still quietly and calmly is extremely important but widely overlooked. The late French philosopher Pascal said: "All the misery of men comes from man's inability to sit quietly in the room, closing his eyes and doing nothing." Coaches teach athletes how to move. They do not teach athletes how to be still. Some Olympic coaches protect their athletes from the disturbing stimuli of the Olympic Village by taking the athlete, a day before the competition to a quiet, pleasant hotel room. They forget that no matter how quiet the room is, the athlete's mind may remain noisy.

Besides sitting still steadily, practicing a few yoga postures will help you gain more control over your body. I suggest practicing the Forward Bend Posture and the Modified Sitting Forward Bend Posture (described in Chapter 5) after sitting still steadily. (But remember you can choose any yoga posture for this purpose.) Learning sitting still is very important. You can move to the next step only after mastering sitting still and calming your body.

BREATH AWARENESS (CONTROL) THROUGH YOGA BREATHING EXPERIENCES

After learning sitting still steadily and calming your body, the next step is learning to control your breath – breath awareness. This is an extremely important technique. I mentioned in the introduction that yoga was instrumental in healing my life and later in my sport career. It was breath awareness and breathing exercises which made me realize that I could control my mind, my mental state, and emotions. Breath is the bridge between the body and mind.

Yoga breathing is a powerful tool. However, you must realize that it also can be harmful if used improperly. As a young boy without guidance, I tried to practice all the Pranayama exercises I found in different yoga books. I realized later that advanced Pranayama exercises can be learned only with the help of qualified instructors.

The breathing exercises in this book can be practiced safely by following the instructions and are sufficient for achieving your goals. If you want to learn and practice more advanced techniques, look for qualified instructors. Also if you wish to learn more about yoga, I strongly suggest publications by Swami Rama, Spiritual Leader and Founder of the Himalayan Institute of Yoga Science, PA.

EXERCISE

In the sitting still steadily position after stilling, calming your body (body awareness), focus your attention on your breathing. Observe, visualize and mentally follow your smooth, deep diaphragmatic breathing as described in the previous chapter.

As we mentioned before, the ultimate goal of most of the yoga breathing exercises is to regulate the mental state by favorably influencing the nervous system. Yoga breathing techniques facilitate concentration and meditation. Through yoga breathing you will gain conscious control over unconscious activities of the autonomic nervous system.

Changes of mental state, changes of feeling, changes of bodily sensations, and postures are registered immediately in the pattern of breathing. For example, fear and anger produce shallow breathing; sorrow produces uneven, spasmodic breathing. Positive emotions create regular breathing. Every change of mental state is reflected in the breath and also in the body. This is also true in reverse — by changing the breathing pattern we can also alter the emotions.

FOCUSING YOUR ATTENTION

Training your attention is a precondition for concentration. You must learn to pay full attention to what you are doing. Where you are physically, you should also be mentally. Some athletes, instead of fully enjoying rest or sleep, bring their troubles and problems with them to bed. Likewise, some athletes focus their attention elsewhere when they are eating. They load their stomachs mechanically while watching television or reading. As a result, natural feelings of fullness occur later, when they experience sensations of pressure or a heaviness in their stomachs.

The first step in training your attention is to practice giving your full attention to each of your daily affairs. For example, when studying, become fully absorbed. When resting, enjoy it fully. When you practice your sport, do it with full attention.

Attention can be involuntary, which means that it is based primarily on reflex. When you reflexively attend to something, it occurs spontaneously and does not require effort. For example, when you hear a fire truck's siren, you may immediately look to see where it is coming from, without thinking about it. Voluntary attention, on the other hand, requires self-discipline. By your own will or effort, you voluntarily direct your attention toward an object or idea. Voluntary attention requires determination and practice.

Self-discipline means that you pay full voluntary attention to what you are doing. Determine to do everything with full attention. Continued attention will lead you to concentration—that is, to keeping focused on the task at hand.

The human mind tends to wander rapidly. Concentrative analyses of top athletes' performances (see Chapter 16) demonstrate how overpowering mental thoughts can be, especially in stressful situations. It is difficult for an athlete to maintain focus without learning to control and calm the mind.

My students start their warm-up (for training and competition) with sitting still steadily and concentrating on breathing, and in addition, for practicing attention and concentration, they usually pick one or two yoga asanas as a part of their warm-up routine, and concentrate fully as they execute it.

Although these exercises take only 2 to 5 minutes, athletes find them useful in shifting themselves from the usual state of awareness to a more focused concentrative state. The exercises serve to get the athlete mentally attuned for the upcoming practice or competition.

DEVELOPING CONCENTRATION

The fourth step on the road to mind control is concentration. Concentration is the most important mental skill, and means fully attending to the task at hand—focusing attention on what you are doing. Lack of concentration is the main reason that athletes' minds wander.

Two important thoughts cannot be held in the mind at the same time. If you concentrate on one negative thought, you cannot at the same time concentrate on the task at hand. Lack of concentration is largely responsible for negative thinking and is the main reason behind all mental errors. If you are distracted by negative or irrelevant thoughts, you cannot concentrate on those things that you need to do to win.

Body and breath awareness exercises described in the previous steps will heighten your concentration. Concentration should be passive and effortless. It should be attained without trying or judging—just allow yourself into a relaxed state of attention focus.

The only way to increase your attention skills and minimize distracting thoughts is to practice. Practice body and breath awareness regularly. The most effective way to improve your concentration is meditation which we will discuss later.

CONCENTRATION DURING COMPETITION

Keeping the mind focused under the high pressure that occurs during a competition is not an easy task. The mind constantly wanders. During a tournament many athletes are not concentrating on the present; their mind might go back to the past—with such thoughts as, "I lost against him once before and I might lose now"—or to the future—thinking about the result of the performance and the consequences of that result. Most athletes think too much during competition and try too hard to control their movements. Emotions, worry, and concern about the result are serious obstacles to concentration.

Concentrative analyses of top athletes' performances when they did their worst illustrate the wide range of thoughts and worries that they underwent. They were shocked when they realized what they were actually thinking about during an important competition (see Chapter 16).

The crucial situations in a competition are the nonaction phases—the moments before, between, and after the actions. Examples of this would be micropauses between touchés in fencing, or waiting for the opponent to serve in tennis. During these moments, the mind can and does wander, and a variety of thoughts occur.

Regular daily practice of concentration will increase your ability to concentrate on the task at hand even under the high pressure of a competition. As I mentioned earlier, most athletes I have worked with have found concentration on breathing and meditation with a mantra to be the preferred exercises to help develop concentration. One of the most effective means for increasing your ability to concentrate is meditation. Athletes claim increased focus and alertness as a result of practicing meditation. Again, the preferred object of meditation is a mantra.

During the competition you must control your thought or your thought will control you. A successful performance (game, match, bout) requires focus on the task at hand—on one touch, game, etc., at a time. You should have a race or game (competition) plan, a performance routine to enhance your concentration and your performance. This will provide you with a framework (time table) of specific things to focus on.

You already learned in Chapter 9, that you are not your thoughts and emotions. You can choose what to relate to. You also learned that you can control many things during the competition, like thoughts, emotions, self-talk, muscle tension, game, routine, responses, and attention focus.

For example, a fencer who is in control observes his or her opponent's actions, moves, automatic responses, habits, weak and strong sides, and intentions in a totally focused way. He or she analyzes the bout situation. The opponent's moves become signals for him and immediately a responding action follows. Then he or she "lets go" of the executed action mentally and re-focuses again.

In some other sport, you may focus your attention—concentrate—on an object that works for you, and stick with it. If your sport is tennis, golf, baseball, basketball, or football, the object of concentration might be the ball. Choosing the ball as your object of concentration might mean focusing your attention on the sight of the ball during its movement. You may also want to concentrate on the sound of the ball when you are hitting, shooting, catching, or passing. As well, you can concentrate on the feeling that you experience physically when you hit, shoot, or catch the ball.

I suggest breathing as a universal object of concentration. This can enhance any sport—golf, basketball, baseball, tennis, football, fencing, and martial arts, as well as sports such as skiing and swimming. Using breathing as an object of concentration means focusing on the flow of breath, on the inhalation and exhalation. You may shift your mind onto your breathing during the nonaction phases of the competition in order to maintain mental focus. (Breathing is also a helpful tool in combating anxiety, which plays a big part during tournaments, and which can cause your mind to wander.)

Because concentration is ultimately sport specific and individual specific, individually tailored autogenic phrases, described and discussed in Chapter 15, are very effective in keeping your focus on the task at hand. With a little work—work that can be very interesting and that will reveal a lot of your inner workings—you can develop some of these simple phrases for yourself. These phrases occupy your mind, thus keeping it from wandering from the present moment. Your object of concentration can be a combination of breathing and your individually tailored autogenic phrases. In all sports, breathing is an important and effective means of refocusing, centering, and regaining and maintaining mental balance.

Concentrative analysis of performances showed that athletes many times need just to be more conscious of things, thoughts, and self-talk they use when performing their best and to use cues to trigger their focus of attention.

Be aware of:

- Focusing on one thing at the critical moment.
- Focusing and being always in the present.
- Not dwelling on your mistakes.
- Developing the ability of selectively attending to critical clues.

SUMMARY

From the previous chapters you learned how to use yoga asanas for different purposes and the four basic steps on the road to self-control. These four basic steps—body awareness (control), breath awareness (control), developing attention, and concentration—lead to meditation and ultimately to self-control.

The exercises of these steps, as well as the asanas described in the previous chapters, are not difficult. It is more difficult to make the commitment and to practice regularly than to execute the exercises.

It is necessary to be aware that only regular practice will produce the desired effect. Even the most effective yoga exercise or mental skill cannot produce any effect without regular practice. For example, muscle dysbalance due to "one-sided" training cannot be corrected if you practice only once a week for a few seconds. These few seconds or minute of practice against hundreds of hours is insignificant and the result is zero! Similarly, you will not solve your weight problem or high cholesterol problem by taking once a week a low-calorie healthy breakfast. The occasional use of any excellent technique is pointless in avoiding heart attack, stroke, or high blood pressure. You need to practice daily and regularly.

In yoga, the essence is, in fact, to develop a more healthier lifestyle—transformation. The "big secret" of yoga is that it changes and normalizes the incorrect way of life. Yoga exercises can be effective only if you practice them regularly and in such duration that it can compensate (balance) the negative effect of an unnatural way of life which became a general lifestyle. Yoga body postures and exercises were developed to supplement and balance (compensate) the one-sided lifestyle.

From the athlete's aspect, yoga is very significant. I observed during many years of working with athletes that yoga is the most effective means for accomplishing the daily practice of concentration (mental skills). Discussion with athletes showed that yoga motivated them the most for developing the habit of practicing mental skills regularly.

Incorporating the basic exercises of the four steps described into your warm-up and/or warm-down routine, mental skill training will become your regular daily routine, a "lifestyle."

The most remarkable thing about yoga is that besides all the mentioned benefits practicing yoga feels good. Athletes claim that after whatever hard training they've done, yoga re-energizes the mind and body.

11

MEDITATION

There are many styles of Meditation. I suggest Maharishi Mahesh Yogi's Transcendental Meditation (TM). More than 500 scientific research studies conducted at 210 universities in more than 30 countries proved the effectiveness of TM. Also my personal experiences with TM as well as studying my athletes' mental preparation strongly support TM.*

The philosophy of TM is based on the concept that just as matter has the potentiality of creating different amounts or levels of energy (gravitational, chemical, and nuclear), thought likewise has the potentiality of creating different amounts or levels of energy.

At progressively finer and more fundamental layers of matter there is more potential energy available. The philosophy of TM holds that as one experiences finer or more abstract layers of thought, the energy and creative intelligence progressively become greater. Maharishi holds that the quality of any action of an individual is directly dependent upon the quality of that individual's thought; that is, if an individual is able to appreciate thought at a finer level and therefore use more thought or mental potentiality, he or she will act with greater efficiency, creativity, and clarity. Maharishi states that by systematically and regularly contacting the field of maximum potentiality, the essential constituent of all fields of existence which is the source of thought, an individual can unfold full mental and creative potentialities. The process of systematic contact with the source of thought is called TM. Maharishi describes TM as follows: "The technique may be defined as turning the attention inward towards

---

* I would like to express appreciation to Mr. Richard LaMarita, who introduced me to TM.

197

the subtle levels of a thought until the mind transcends the experience of the subtlest state of the thought and arrives at the source of thought."

TM is a very specific technique different from other styles of meditation. The process is unlike other systems of meditation since it is effortless, easy, and does not involve any concentration, contemplation, or any type of physical or mental control. In fact, effortlessness is the very key to its effectiveness.

Most systems of meditation claim that the tendency of the mind is to wander, and in order to bring it into contact with the source of thought the mind must first be controlled. To achieve this control, rigorous discipline is used both during the meditation and during preparation for meditation. According to Maharishi, the tendency of the mind is not to wander aimlessly, but to move naturally in the direction of experiences that bring greater happiness and enjoyment. The experience of increasingly finer aspects of thought is progressively more enjoyable. Therefore, one only needs to know how to begin to experience finer aspects of thoughts, and spontaneously the attention is drawn inward until it transcends to the source of thought. The technique involves no suggestion, belief, mental control, or physical manipulation.

Unlike other systems of meditation and personal development, there are no constraints on the individual's diet and daily habits. Maharishi emphasizes that TM is practiced as a preparation for successful activity and not as an escape from the problems of life. He states that by spending 20 minutes twice each day in contacting the source of thought, the individual develops his or her full potential.

TM uses a mantra, but you are not asked to focus upon it. A mantra is a vehicle to draw the mind back to its own source, a reservoir of energy, creativity, and intelligence. It is practiced sitting comfortably with eyes closed for 20 minutes twice a day—once in the morning and once in the afternoon. It can be done anywhere—at home, on an airplane, on the train, in your office. When you begin to meditate, use the thinking process with the mantra as a medium in the precise but restful way you have been taught.

As the mind settles down, it naturally grows in creativity, intelligence, and energy. The deepest level of the mind is the field of maximum energy and intelligence. Here we locate an unbound reservoir of pure energy and creative intelligence. From here all thoughts arise. This is the source of thought. The source of thought is the field of pure consciousness.

A level of awareness where consciousness is open to itself, awake to its full potential. It is silent, yet ready to function with maximum dynamism, clarity, and orderliness. After 20 minutes of practice you can plunge into activity, rested, and rejuvenated with more creativity and intelligence.

TM is easy to learn and enjoyable to practice. You will experience the benefits of TM immediately and they accumulate over time. TM is easy to understand; it is simple, natural, and effortless.

Through TM we can achieve the extension of the range of your normal faculties to their maximum possible value, a level of development rarely experienced by most individuals.

The TM program is safe and effective; it can be systematically and uniformly taught and is quick to give results. Moreover, all of these features can be demonstrated objectively.

TM is an effortless, simple process, but it requires a qualified instructor. It cannot be learned from a book. The reason for this is that individuals respond in slightly different ways to the initial stages of the experience, which is a novel one, and instructions must be adjusted on the basis of subjective reports so that the process will continue easily. This can only be accomplished effectively through the personal presence of a trained teacher (to understand this point better, you need only imagine the difficulty of teaching someone to dream—in the state of consciousness that had never been experienced before—by means of written description alone.).

At the end of this chapter you will find the address and location of the TM centers in North America. Call or write the one that is closest to you.

A TM course takes four consecutive days of two-hour classes, after a preparatory lecture and interview. The investment will be probably the best one you ever had.

THOUGHT: ACHIEVEMENT AND ENEMY

Thought is the basis of any activity. A project, a bridge, a monument, an airplane, each began as a thought. Your goal, training, and game (race) plan starts with your thought. Thought is the basis of action which is the basis of achievement. But as you will learn from the concentrative analyses of athletes worst performances (and I am sure also from your own personal experience), if your thought is negative it can be your biggest enemy, destroying your confidence, concentration, and performance. The clearer, more creative, and more intelligent your thoughts are, the more successful your design, action, and performance will be.

Thoughts, like waterfalls, are pouring constantly in your mind. We experience thousands of thoughts every day. We recognize them as a picture, word, an idea or an emotion.

Normally, you are aware of a thought all at once in its fully developed form. But thoughts do not arise fully developed. They come from a field, existing at some abstract, more subtle level before becoming totally clear.

TM deals directly with the activity of the mind—thinking. It is basically a procedure for experiencing the mechanics of the thinking process in a new direction. As I already mentioned, normally you are aware of a thought in its fully developed form. There must be prior stages in the development of all thought. It is possible to bring these stages to conscious awareness in a systematic way. (See Table 8.)

The mind is like the ocean. A thought starts from the deepest level of the ocean of the mind. The surface level is the conscious mind. Thoughts start on the deepest level like a bubble starts at the ocean's bottom. As the bubble rises, it becomes progressively larger until it surfaces and is recognized consciously as a bubble (or thought). It rises through the entire depth of consciousness. The point being that through the practice of TM the thought bubble could be appreciated through all the levels of consciousness and not just at the surface level, thereby expanding the power of the conscious mind manyfold, i.e., as your consciousness transcends all the way to the bottom, it has reached the source of all creative intelligence.

TM uses thought associated with a "sound" for this purpose (the reasons for it is explained in terms of the structure of subjective sensory experience), called "mantra." There are a particular set of sounds (mantras) handed down for centuries which have the special property of becoming increasingly euphonious and pleasing as they are perceived at prior stages. The ancient tradition has presented not only these sounds (mantras), but also a system of rules or formulas by which they are to be assigned to individuals. The idea being that a particular sound has a capacity that resonates best with the structure of a particular nervous system.

There are three states of consciousness: sleeping, dreaming, and waking. Knowledge is different in different states of consciousness (sleep

		Mind	Body
Relative State always changing (R)	Sleeping	Little Activity	Decreased metabolic rate 8-15%
	Dreaming	Some Activity	Some rest
	Waking	Activity	Active
Absolute State It is what is is (A)	Transcendental, pure conscious- ness	Quiet, still, not active, at the same time restful alertness	Decreased Metabolic rate 18-25% Restful alertness

Table 7: Stages of Conscious Awareness

—illusion, waking—cause and effect). Sleeping, dreaming and waking states are relative (R) states because they are changing.

TM produces a fourth state of consciousness: transcendental or pure consciousness. It is an absolute (A) state. (See Table 7.)

TM incorporates all states. When we meditate, we go to the (A) level.

A fourth state of consciousness is introduced during transcendental meditation. It is is a higher, unique state. During TM we experience it as transcendental pure consciousness—no thoughts, no mantra, just pure consciousness. Pure consciousness is always present between thoughts—a small gap in between thoughts, only we are not aware of it.

With practicing TM we gradually expand transcendental conscious-ness, not only during TM, but we also expand it in all our thoughts and daily activities. TM is a process of systematic purification of the nervous system, leading to a continually clearer experience of the fourth state of consciousness (transcendental—pure consciousness) and then to a fifth state wherein pure consciousness is maintained along with waking, dreaming, and sleeping.

This fifth state of consciousness is "enlightenment." For centuries, the term enlightenment has been a vague expression of a level of purity, integration, and personal growth possessed by only a few.

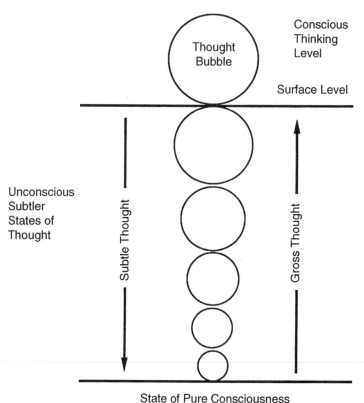

Thought Bubble

Conscious Thinking Level

Surface Level

Unconscious Subtler States of Thought

Subtle Thought

Gross Thought

State of Pure Consciousness
Source of Creative Intelligence

Table 8: Levels of Thought   Created by Patricia Drake Hemingway

Maharishi has for the first time clearly defined and described the state of "enlightenment." Enlightenment is identical with the fifth state of consciousness. In this state, pure consciousness is stabilized and integrated with waking activity, dreaming, and deep sleep.

There are specific criteria in terms of subjective experience as well as specific criteria in terms of physiological measurement.

Gaining cosmic enlightenment it is permanent. It is a life with true freedom. Being completely free, applying full potential in all of our activities, we have more skill, more self-assurance, self-content with inner happiness. You begin to live 200 percent (100 percent inner, 100 percent outer).

To learn more about TM I suggest three very good publications:

Hemmingway, Patricia Drake. *The Transcendental Meditation Primer: How To Stop Tension and Start Living*. New York: Dell Publishing Co., Inc.

Denniston, Denise.*The TM Book How To Enjoy The Rest Of Your Life*. Fairfield, Iowa: Fairfield Press.

Roth, Robert. *Maharishi Mahesh Yogi's TM*. New York: Donald L. Fine

For more analytical reading, I suggest:

The collected papers *Scientific Research On The TM Program*, Maharishi European Research University Press

TM TO INCREASE YOUR PERFORMANCE

Athletes are exposed to stress much more than the average individual. Besides the everyday stress from work, study, family, and personal problems, top athletes have tremendous daily training loads which both physically and mentally exhaust the body. Another source of stress overload comes from the high pressure to produce constantly top results, from stressful competitions, and from the anxiety of losing and its consequences.

TM offers many benefits to athletes. With regular practice, athletes can release stress; that is, the nervous system will be stronger, more flexible, and free of stress. Research studies also show that TM is the most effective technique for releasing stress and inducing deep rest. In TM, after a few minutes the body's metabolic rate decreases 18-25 percent. During sleep, the metabolic rate decreases only after 5-6 hours and only 15 percent.

The high training load, the pressure of competition, joy of victory, agony of defeat, anxiety about losing, etc., make athletes very emotional, experiencing a rollercoaster of moods and emotions. Practicing TM twice daily in the morning and in the afternoon, athletes get deep rest, the tension is released from the body, and the body will be rejuvenated. The nervous system is purified. Energy is accumulating.

Our thoughts can be clear, creative, and intelligent, or less creative, unclear, and negative. Negative thoughts are the biggest enemy of athletes. Sports psychology is dealing with this topic very intensively. Positive thinking, substituting negative thoughts with positive ones, focus of attention on your race, game plans—on the task at hand, etc.—are effective techniques. TM goes to the root, to the source of thought.

Thoughts come from the field of pure energy deep within the mind, existing in some abstract, more subtle level before becoming totally clear or "negative."

Your thoughts will be more powerful, creative, and intelligent if you contact the reservoir of energy and intelligence through TM. Every thought has some kind of intelligent purpose or direction. We have thousands of thoughts every day which need energy. Each thought has some direction which needs creativity. All thoughts, as we usually experience them, are directed outward through thinking and speech (self-talk) and then into action.

During TM we use a vehicle, a specific thought called a mantra. Because of the nature of the vehicle and the way we are thought to experience it, the mind automatically goes within, following the thought of the mantra back to the source of all thought to the field of pure energy, deep in the mind, experiencing the process of transcendental (pure) consciousness. As a result of this process your thoughts will be more powerful, clear, creative, and intelligent.

Here I want to point out another aspect. All the athletes' activities require effort, concentration, focus of attention, and physical and mental control. The mental skills and techniques also require some kind of control, concentration, and suggestions. Athletes are overwhelmed with effort, suggestions, and control. TM, as an effortless, natural, technique without any kind of control, suggestions, and concentration, is a good compensation and supplement to an athlete's program and life.

Athletes report being more rested, and having more energy from TM. Further reports show better concentration, having clearer thoughts and experiencing less stress.

Research studies (TM related to sport) show faster reaction time, superior perceptual motor performance, increased speed, improvement in speed, accuracy actions and improvement in athletic performances. TM increases endurance, the ability to hold up — to maintain peak performance for the very end of a game, match or race and TM enables us to refine our thoughts.

All our activity is based on thoughts. If we can tap the origin of our thoughts, we tap the origin of our creative intelligence. By practicing TM regularly over a period of time, athletes can realize and use their full potential not only in sport, but also in their private lives.

How do you incorporate TM into your sport preparation? Should TM substitute other mental skills?

TM is not a substitute for any mental skills or training activities. TM is an effective, natural, beneficial addition to your sport training as well as to your everyday life activities. TM is a means of preparation for your sport and daily activities.

You meditate for 20 minutes in the morning before you start your training or daily activities, and 20 minutes again in the afternoon (or early evening) before your evening activity begins. These two TM sessions will provide you with renewed energy and prepare you for the activity ahead, producing more physical and mental energy, more clarity and creativity in thought, and higher productivity.

As a result of practicing TM regularly you will notice a general improvement in all areas of your activity, like better relation, and interaction with your coach and team mates (as well as fellow workers); more clarity, creativity, and intelligence in all of your thoughts and actions; and expanded awareness. You will notice that you perceive things around you with greater sharpness of mind, and more sensitivity to your own feelings and desires. You will notice more energy and enthusiasm for your activity, that you are able to stay calm under pressure, and the ability to be more open and flexible in your approaches to achieving your goals. You will also notice improvement in mental skills.

12

THE POWER OF AWARENESS IN SPORTS AND LIFE

Awareness significantly affects all aspects of your life from your everyday activities and sport performance to the process of healing and aging. We usually undervalue and do not use its power.

You cannot control what you are not aware of. Many times athletes improve their performances by simply being aware of, for example, muscle tension in the shoulders when serving in tennis or thrusting in fencing.

Your awareness plays an important role in explaining what is happening in your body. As Deepak Chopra, M.D., pointed out in his best-selling book *Ageless Body, Timeless Mind*, "The biochemistry of the body is a product of awareness. Beliefs, thoughts, and emotions create chemical reactions that uphold life in every cell." Each thought, feeling and belief has an effect on your performance as well as on your healing and aging process, directly or indirectly. There is no mind body separation; mind and body are one. One influences the other.

Fear, anxiety, and doubt can destroy your performance, your many years of sports preparation. Depression weakens your immune system. A memory of a lost bout, a defeat, or a thought of failure releases the same destructive hormones as the actual stress itself.

Your sports performance, healing and aging are complex processes. They are not only physical, but also mental. You can change your sports performance as well as your aging or healing process by what you think, believe, and feel.

It has always been fascinating to me to observe how my fencers could compete well in one bout, producing excellent results, and in the next one compete poorly. In such a short time the fitness level and technique could not change so significantly to affect the performance. This phenomenon can be attributed to a shift in awareness of belief, thought, and emotions.

Similar shifts in awareness, describes Chopra, also occur in spontaneous cures of cancer, healing, and aging processes. "Research on spontaneous cures of cancer has shown that just before the cure appears almost every patient experiences a dramatic shift in awareness." The patient knows that he or she will be healed like the athlete who knows he or she will succeed.

The body is metabolizing everything we see, hear, smell, and touch even if we are not aware of it. If you feel happy or depressed, every cell in your body will learn it and be affected.

Happiness, joy, and love strengthen your immune system. Anxiety and depression can manifest as ulcers or spasms. The body projects thoughts; it mirrors any mental event.

Athletes many times read their opponent's mind from their body language, gestures, and facial expressions.

Studies show that fencers who believe in victory win more bouts and tend to fence more actively. A fencer's belief in victory has a direct correlation with the percentage of winning bouts. Belief in victory also has a relationship with how a fencer behaves during the bout and has a direct correlation with active fencing. Active fencing means taking the initiative. The active fencer makes things happen in the bout.

Other studies have been done comparing fencing action in important bouts under high pressure with less important bouts under less pressure. In less important bouts, the relationship between belief in victory and attacks was not statistically significant but demonstrated a tendency toward becoming significant. In important bouts, however, this relationship is significantly increased.

Awareness and attention can significantly increase your performance and make your sports preparation more effective.

Exercises in the chapters on self-study, and autogenic training use the power of awareness and attention to alter and control involuntary function, to demonstrate and to convince that relaxed intention (passive attention) automatically tends to realize and seeks fulfillment. For example, the balloon, the closed-eye, and the pendulum exercises (see Chapter 9) demonstrate how an intention enervates a certain muscle group, generates impulses in the nervous system and produces unconscious muscular activity, or they demonstrate how a voluntary action can be inhibited by intention. The heaviness, warmth, cold and heartbeat exercises (see Chapter 9), as well as the autogenic basic exercises, demonstrate the ability to control involuntary functions.

Studies of ideo-motor training showed that perfect execution of a sports skill, a perfect performance does not depend only on the technique, and fitness, but also on what the athlete focuses on.

Studies with ideo-motor set-up proved that the attention focus the athlete holds in mind about the movement greatly influences the structure of the movement. This attention focus (ideo-motor set-up) is a psychological factor that relates to movement. It is one of the main elements in determining the form of your movement and perfecting it.

Studies showed that the athlete's focus during performance is of crucial importance in determining the actual form of the movement. If the athlete changes the area of focus, he or she will change the structure of the movement and modify the technique. Examples include the long jump, triple jump, gymnastics, and fencing.

There are two different types of ideomotoric setups in sport. The ideomotoric set-ups can vary, depending on the type of sport and situation which is called for. One is called a stable, or fixed ideomotoric setup (IS) and the other is a changing, or variable IS. The stable IS is typical in sports where the movements do not change, and where the competitive conditions are relatively stable. Examples of fixed, or stable set-ups involve movements such as the high jump, long jump, diving, shot put, gymnastics and archer. A stable IS creates a readiness in the athlete, and tunes him or her up by focusing the mind and body on the specific movement.

The variable ideomotoric setup is used in sports in which the athlete must respond to a rapidly changing environment. The stimuli can come from either the athlete's own movement against a changing terrain (such as in skiing), or an opponent responding to the athlete's movements (as in tennis, fencing, or wrestling). The changing ideomotoric setup is a type of plan, or model for solving the athlete's situation. The objective is to maximize performance by activating all of the athlete's past experiences and current skills.

The ideomotoric setup is a psychological factor that relates to movement. It is one of the main elements in determining the form of your movement and perfecting it. The image which the athlete holds in mind about the movement greatly influences the structure of the movement.

The sensory content of the ideomotoric setup-that is, the sensations that the athlete focuses on during the performance-is of crucial importance in determining the actual form of the movement. If the athlete changes the area of focus (through the ideomotoric setup), he or she will change the structure of the movement and modify the technique.

This phenomenon has been studied extensively in Eastern Europe, The researchers Djachkov, Geremin, Ceresnevova and Tishler (1965) demonstrated the importance of the ideomotoric setup by studying the effects of ideomotoric setups in different sports. For example, long and triple jumpers were given the test of using two different types of ideomotoric setups. The athletes alternated between the two set-ups during practice. The set-ups were:

- To focus on the strength of the jumper's take off,
- To focus on the speed with which the jumper approached the jumping point.

The study demonstrated that changing the athlete's ideomotoric set-up led to differences in the athlete's performances; insofar as time, place in and strength factors were concerned. The ideomotoric mental setup which focused on the strength of the takeoff created an active, pulling movement of the body. The setup which focused on speed of the approach run created a reactive, explosive movement. The overall execution of an action requiring both speed and strength depends not only on the athlete's physical ability, but also on his or her mental setup.

Similar results were achieved when studying the effect of the mental set-up in gymnastic vaulting. In this experiment, Ceresnevova gave the gymnasts two tasks when executing the vault, to either focus on the speed of their takeoffs or on the height of the vault. The athletes concentrating on a swift takeoff not only produced high vaults, but more coordinated movements overall than when focusing on the height of the vault alone. Once again, demonstrating that what the athlete focuses about on during the performance can have a great impact on their results.

Yet another example of using IT as a mental set-up involved athletes in the task of a vertical jump. The athletes had to jump down from a platform, and then immediately had to jump as high as they could. As the height of the platform was increased, the height of the athletes' upward jump after landing was decreased. This was true for all mental setups. However, the setups affected how quickly the athletes started their upwards jumps. When concentrating on speed the athletes started upward more quickly than when using the other setups. The focus on speed, rather than strength again made a positive difference.

An important conclusion that is drawn from this research: for all speed and strength movements, the best mental setup is not on strength, but speed. In the cases of long jumping, triple jump, gymnastic vaulting, and vertical jump, focusing on speed rather than power or strength creates the best performances.

ADAPTING THE MENTAL SET-UP TO THE ATHLETE'S LEVEL OF SKILL

The appropriate mental set-up also depends upon the athlet's individual skill level and experience. A mental set-up which is effective for a top athlete may not be effective for a beginner or middle level athlete - and vice versa.

This phenomenon has been studied in Eastern Europe. In a study, Tishler looked into the amount of time that fencers require to complete a "direct attack." Fencers were timed from the beginning of their movement, until the completed execution of a head cut with fleche and lunge.

In this study the fencers were given the test of trying a number of different mental set-ups as they executed their fencing moves. At first, the fencers were all required to complete a direct attack without using any mental set-up. Next, each fencer was asked to execute the attack using one of four different mental set-ups. With each mental set up the action was repeated three times. The four mental set-ups included:

- Focusing on the start of the movement of the fencer's front leg-making an explosive movement with the front leg.
- Focusing on the start of an explosive take off with the back leg.

- Focusing on coordination or the "synchrony" of movements of both legs.

- Focusing on the speed of movement of the arm (with weapon)-to hit the target as quickly as possible without attempting to control the movement of the legs.

The lower level and middle level fencers performed the fastest attacks, with mental set-ups which focused on leg movement. That is, they did best with the first three mental set-ups. The technical level of these fencers required them to focus on the take off-and the factors related to the take off. When these fencers focused on the speed of their arm movement (the last mental set-up), the takeoffs, were late, and errors occurred in hand-foot coordination.

The opposite was true for top level fencers. Focusing on the takeoff from the front leg or back leg actually decreased the effectiveness of their attacks. When the fencers focused on coordinating their leg movements, they had the same results as when they had no mental set-up at all. However, when the top level fencers, focused on the speed of their arm movements they increased the effectiveness and speed of their attacks. For these fencers, focusing on arm speed improved all aspects of the take-off, and increased the overall speed of the attack.

Thus, demonstrating that the advanced fencers increased their speed and effectiveness of their attacks using different a mental setup, than lower level fencers. Presumably, this difference was due to the fact that top level fencers had so mastered their leg movement that there was no need to think about or concentrate on the legs, just on the speed of the arm holding the weapon.

Yoga teaches that consciousness creates the body. Awareness and attention have the power to alter the body. As Chopra noted, "The human brain changes its thoughts into thousands of chemicals every second. The body matches the mind; it moves with thoughts."

If you decide that you want something, if you set a goal, your body responds to achieve your goal; the intention triggers the response. Awareness is a field of energy, a big power, but it can also work against you.

The most important means for influencing and programming awareness is belief.

The quality of your sports performance and ultimately your life depends on the quality of you attention and intention. Use the power of attention to your benefit.

Now that you are aware of the power of awareness, use these techniques for influencing your involuntary nervous system to your advantage.

- Practice TM two times daily for 20 minutes.

TM develops a settled, deep, restful state and releases stress. This can be the foundation for your daily training, and work activities as well as for healing and aging processes.

The most basic rhythm of nature is activity and rest. This is also the most important principle of sports training.

TM is also a powerful healing technique. TM produces a deep, relaxed state which is the precondition for any healing process, for curing any disorders as well as for practicing mental skills like imagery or concentration.

TM affects the aging process. Studies show that after five or more years of daily practice, the practitioner appears to be 12 years younger than their actual age..

TM unites the thinking mind with its source with pure energy, awareness.

- Be in touch with nature.

If your sport requires practicing indoors, make sure that you find some time to practice outdoors as well. Practice your supplemental sports or exercises outdoors like running, swimming, skiing, games, etc. Plan your vacations to be outdoors and enjoy walking in the forest, basking in the sun, enjoying activities in nature. Take at least a few minutes every day to walk in the park, to look at the sky, to notice a beautiful flower or a blossoming tree. Become aware of the beauty of nature, enjoy it at least for a moment.

Nature is a healer. Lie on the grass, look at the sky and at the clouds, feel the warmth of the sun, take a few deep breaths whenever you can. Pay conscious attention to your bodily functions. Be aware that every one of your involuntary functions can be consciously controlled.

- Allow the free flow of energy, prana, in your body.

According to yoga, our essential nature is a flow of energy called prana. The main source of prana is breathing. Making your breathing slow, regular, and fluent assures regular circulation of prana in your body. Pay attention to proper breathing and practice regularly.

Another source of prana is food. Eat fresh fruits, vegetables, and healthy and nutritious meals. Drink pure spring water and juice. Have a proper eating regime, do not eat in a rush.

Aside from practicing your sport competitively, focus also on the harmonious development of your body. Practice yoga supplemental, regenerational and yoga corrective exercises. Have fun and pleasure; enjoy your physical activity. Keep in mind that your brain changes your thoughts into thousands of chemicals every second. Your body matches your mind.

- Avoid negative emotions

Thoughts like fear, anger, etc. poison your body, increase your aging process, make you less beautiful, and decrease the flow of energy, prana.

- Avoid stress, conflicted behavior, and violence.

Instead, cultivate positive emotions such as love, joy, friendship and happiness that produce "good" hormones, "good" body chemistry, decrease your aging process, and increase the flow of prana.

What is happening to you is a result of how you perceive yourself. If you want to change your performance, change your awareness first. If you want to change your body, change your awareness first.

- Perception influences awareness.

Awareness is a learned phenomenon. All of us have different perceptions of anything. If you are sad or depressed, you see everything differently from when you are happy.

If you start your bout or game with the awareness and thought, "I lost against this guy before; I might lose again," or with the thought, "I practiced good and hard. I beat this guy before; I will beat him again," your body will metabolize your thought accordingly. Your body knows how you feel about yourself.

Coaches used to say to athletes that it is not the stress, the conditions and pressure, but how you respond to it that is important. External events can not hurt you. Only when and how you interpret it will or can hurt you.

Modern pentathlon athletes who compete in five different sports—swimming, running, shooting, horseback riding and fencing—know very well that each of the five sports requires a different awareness. Research with modern pentathlon athletes showed that in fencing those athletes achieved the best results who had a "cold anger," who "saw" their opponents as adversaries. In shooting, however, a settled, relaxed mind set produced the best results.

Awareness, attention, and intention are closely connected. When practicing, follow the following guidelines:

- Be certain and confident; do not doubt the outcome of your intention.
- Do not be anxious about the result. Have a nonstriving attitude.
- Your intention should be specific and definite.
- Have a non-interference, "Let it happen," attitude without striving or evaluating the process.
- Do not pay attention to details of the process involved.

These steps will help you practice awareness:

- Sit comfortably and relax your body.
- Induce the sensation of total calmness.
- Intend the outcome you want. Be specific.
- Visualize the outcome and/or repeat it in your mind.
- Do not force; concentrate! Your intention should be natural, like walking or raising your hand.
- Expect and believe in the outcome; do not doubt it!
- Know that it is certain!

- Be aware that doubt, worry, and attachment will lead to failure.
- Eliminate attachment; use feedback.

13 ▬▬▬▬

THE POWER OF SUGGESTION

All our life consists of suggestion. Our mothers and fathers started to talk to us on the day we were born. We learned from our caring parents constantly; we received suggestions from our teachers. A coach gives suggestions to his or her athletes; friends, teammates and fellow workers are always trying to convince us of their ideas and we respond to them.

Transference of an idea or thought to another person is usually done by dialogue. Another way of transferring thought is by suggestion. Our point is to make the transference of thought in the most effective way.

You can make your dialogue more effective if you speak in shorter sequences and do not use more than three sentences. Remember that the attention focus of your partner is limited. He or she usually pays attention to your first sentences, then starts to think about the answer. On the other hand, you will be more aware of your last sentences if you speak for a long time, and your impression of your partner's response will be inaccurate. Talking in short sentences, two or three at a time, enables fast, adequate communication.

Emotional states influence your dialogue. Experienced coaches know that after a painful defeat, when someone is upset and emotional, it is better to wait for a while, leaving the athlete alone to calm down, before going into the suggestion or evaluation session.

The most effective way of transference of thought is by suggestion. To make this method effective it is necessary to create a mental state that is suitable for accepting suggestions; we call this state an altered state of consciousness.

What are the conditions for creating such a favorable mental state for accepting suggestions? What is an altered state of consciousness?

We are in a different state of consciousness during the day and night. Each of our activities requires a different level of consciousness, different degrees of brain control. When we involve in sports activity, work or sleep we are in a different state of consciousness. For example, when you relax in the Relaxation Posture your brain activity is decreased, your brain control is "switched off." You feel good because this state reduces fear and anxiety and produces calmness.

A similar "switch-off" occurs when sleeping, during meditation, autogenic training, and also when you are involved in your hobbies. They all have the same goal—to "switch off" the control system of the brain in order to accumulate and regenerate the energy for your following activities.

The external condition for creating an altered state is the elimination of the external distractions and stimuli to enhance concentration, and to create a calm environment (quiet place, relaxed comfortable position, closing the eyes, etc.).

The internal conditions are the narrowing of thoughts, which like a waterfall are pouring into our mind all day long, and the reduction of mental control. For this we use mental devices that help to reduce the brain's activity and narrow our attention focus. The simplest way to achieve it is through repetition of sounds, words or sentences.

You can get to an altered state of consciousness by a "natural way" such as sleeping. Also, the ancient systems of relaxation—yoga, hypnosis, meditation—all serve to achieve this goal.

These principles are the basis of hypnosis, self-hypnosis, and the autogenic training described in detail in this book.

When we get into an altered state of consciousness the brain's activities are reduced, our attention focus is narrowed and we more easily pay attention to a given suggestion and are more receptive to accept it.

My method uses concentrative analysis; the spontaneous self-talk, suggestions we are giving to ourselves when performing our best for creating our suggestions.

Dr. Michael Ben-Menachem, a noted psychologist, suggests using positive past events as a basis for creating suggestions. It is especially helpful for people with low self-esteem.

He suggests keeping a daily diary where you put down at the end of the day the most important things that happened to you during the day.

What did you think about, with whom and what were you talking about? Comment on your work, your studies, etc.

Each recorded activity is then marked with a plus "+" or minus "-" sign depending on how you evaluate it. At the end of the day you add the number of plus and minus events. In the following step he suggests choosing four or five positive events (sentences) which will be the building blocks for creating suggestions.

This method uses the past positive events for creating suggestions, for strengthening the self-confidence and self-esteem.

In the final step you will get into a deep relaxed state; in the middle of this state you will read two times your suggestions, and then, closing your eyes, you will continue to experience relaxation again.

As you will see in learning basic autogenic training, developing an altered state can be used as a base or a vehicle for giving yourself specific suggestions based on your needs.

When you do your best you are in an altered state. Or, as a yogi would say: Your prana is flowing perfectly.

You will learn to use the power of suggestion in the following chapter on autogenic training.

14

SPORT-MODIFIED AUTOGENIC TRAINING*

Autogenic Training (AT) is on of the most important autoregulatory system for athletes used today. Widely used in Eastern Europe, it involves relaxation and concentration. AT is a method which, when practiced regularly, contributes to fast recovery of strength and elimination of the symptoms of stress and restlessness. It also eradicates incorrect habits, negative thoughts, and anxiety, and allows the athlete to achieve the required properties of successful performance. AT allows the athlete to mobilize and use his or her own natural energy and power in order to achieve a definite objective. Through AT, it is possible to influence both the emotions and the functions of the autogenic nervous system.

Even though the idea of controlling autonomic and unconscious functions was, prior to 1960, thought to be impossible in the western world, the phenomena of mind/body self-regulation exhibited by yogis awakened the curiosity and interest of British physicians more than 200 years ago. Later, British and other European physicians began to study the mind/body relationship.

It was around 1910 that Dr. J. Schultz of Germany began to develop a mind-body training system called Autogenic Training (AT), also called self-generated or self-motivated training. Schultz developed AT from hypnosis and yoga. It occurred to him that perhaps hypnosis was unpredictable because the patient often unconsciously resisted the doctor. If patients were able to direct the procedure themselves, with the doctor acting as teacher, they would offer less resistance.

---

* This chapter is taken from the author's book *Clearing the Path to Victory: A Self-Guided Mental Training Program for Athletes.* Counter Parry Press, PA.

Schultz correctly identified some of the effective components of hypnotherapy and yoga and incorporated them into a method of self-regulation. He realized that self-regulation would have to be simple to be effective. Neither hypnosis nor yoga is simple. Hypnosis is especially complex since it requires a psychologist who has developed trust and rapport with the patient. Even then, some individuals resist the process. Schultz therefore drew effective elements from both hypnosis and yoga to create a more practical method than either.

A critical step was taken in the development of AT when Schultz required his patients to record their physical sensations during hypnosis. He learned that the heaviness, warmth in the limbs, calm breathing, slow heart rate, and general relaxation were common to all patients. He inferred that if these sensations could be induced through a methodology, the patient's relaxation would be followed by a state similar to a hypnotic trance. (An actual trance need not be the goal of the procedure; a milder variant resembling self-hypnosis is sufficient.)

This was the basic idea behind Schultz's method, and methods of inducing the desired physical sensations became, along with autosuggestive phrases, standard exercises in AT. The autosuggestive phrases (verbal formulas) are organized into six standard physiologically oriented exercises focusing on heaviness in the extremities, warmth in the extremities, calm and regular heartbeat, calm and regular breathing, the sensation of warmth in the solar plexus, and the sensation of coolness in the forehead. Schultz sought to speed up the calming of the body and nervous system with verbal cues and influences.

Schultz further developed his standard exercises by encouraging patients to heighten or intensify those sensations that occur in the body by concentrating on the sensations. To do so, he utilized classic yoga techniques. Yoga can be seen in many aspects of Schultz's method: muscle relaxation (similar to Savasana), the method of concentration (Raja Yoga), body awareness or proprioception (Laya Yoga), repetition of mantra-like autosuggestive phrases (Mantra Yoga), and closing the eyes, reducing external and internal stimulations (Pratyhara).

THE TWO PRINCIPLES OF AT: RELAXATION AND CONCENTRATION

Two underlying premises of AT are (1) that the human being is a psychosomatic unit (in other words, the body and mind influence each other), and (2) that words, or verbal stimuli, and their accompanying imagery can potentially alter physiological, cognitive, and emotional states. The physiological basis of AT is that a close causal connection exists between the processes of the brain cortex and the autonomic processes (the part of the nervous system that governs involuntary actions).

The following example illustrates the mechanism and effect of AT. If we ask an individual to secrete a certain type of stomach fluid, his response quite naturally is that this is an impossible task because the secretion of stomach fluid is an involuntary process. But if we instruct him to imagine vividly that he is eating a lemon, surprisingly, a natural physiological response is for his stomach to secrete a fluid that it would secrete if he were to eat a lemon. This reaction implies that a conditioned stimulus-response mechanism has developed. The verbal stimulus produces the same response as the actual lemon. The sympathetic and parasympathetic nervous systems have been affected by verbal stimuli and visualization. (Note: The sympathetic and parasympathetic nervous systems are parts of the autonomic nervous system. They are related to secretion, muscle tone, and blood vessel dilation and contraction.)

Essentially, the same physiological mechanism applies in relaxation. The suggestions of heaviness, warmth, and relaxation make the muscles more sensitive, decrease muscle tension, and enhance relaxation. Hence, the essence of AT in Schultz's view is concentrative relaxation: while the muscles of the body are in a completely relaxed state, inner mental activity is focused on determined objectives. This consciously directed mental activity allows greater conscious influence in regulating the various biological processes that before were independent of conscious control.

Psycho-physiologically, AT is based on three main principles: (1) mental repetition of topographically oriented verbal phrases, (2) mental activity known as passive concentration, and (3) reduction of exteroceptive and proprioceptive afferent stimulation. (Note: exteroceptive means activated by stimuli from outside; proprioceptive means activated by stimuli from within. Afferent has to do with conveying impulses toward a nerve center.)

AT has two main components: relaxation and concentration. Relaxation means the release of all muscles. This physical relaxation is the first step toward mental relaxation accompanied by the sensations of harmony and composure. Concentration means attending mentally to a certain image, which then exerts an influence over the entire organism. This influence is enhanced by relaxation. In AT, physiological changes are directed through the focusing of attention.

Concentration during AT is achieved passively, through visualization and imagination. It does not occur through force of will. Goal-directed effort and an active interest are avoided. You do not force concentration in any way; you simply let it happen. Passive concentration occurs when your body is a in a deeply relaxed state but your mind is alert—attention is passively focused on a particular image and on the self-suggestion phrases. These phrases are introduced in Chapters 7, 8, and 13.

Autogenic training optimizes passive attention and helps learning autonomic control through passive attention. In AT you attend passively to certain areas (such as the arms) and speak internally to your body ("My arms are heavy, my arms are warm"). The muscle tension activity will change in the area where your passive attention was focused.

Body control is achieved through passive attention and not active trying, and the important part of the control is the process and the attention to it—not the outcome.

AT implies self-control. The student is responsible for his or her own growth and mental state. No one can make you control yourself. Hence, there is a change in the source of responsibility—it rests with the athlete and no one else.

To summarize, AT involves two principles that interact with each other: relaxation and concentration. Concentration involves focusing on certain images; it is not achieved through force or will power. Passive concentration—the let-it-happen concept—is one of the most important factors in AT. Relaxation and concentration work together to help athletes gain power and control over their bodies, leading to more enjoyment and success in their sports.

SCHULTZ'S CLASSICAL AT

The classical AT of Schultz has six categories of exercise: muscle, blood vessels, heart, breathing, organs of the stomach, and the head. AT is based on an exact system and consists of the following standard exercises, which are paired with complementary autosuggestive phrases.

Classical AT was developed for clinical purposes in psychotherapy, and the training was very slow—commonly 7 to 8 months long. The heaviness exercise was, for instance, practiced one limb at a time, with one week for each limb, and so on through each of the other exercises.

Classical AT Exercises	
Standard exercise	**Auto-suggestion**
1. Heaviness exercise	My right arm is heavy.
	My left arm is heavy.
	My right leg is heavy.
	My left leg is heavy.
	My whole body is heavy.
2. Warmth exercise	My right arm is warm.
	My left arm is warm.
	My right leg is warm.
	My left leg is warm.
	My whole body is warm.
3. Respiration exercise	My breathing is calm.
	I am breathing easily.
4. Cardiac exercise	My heartbeat is strong and quiet.
5. Solar plexus exercise	My solar plexus is warm. Warmth is pouring into the solar plexus.
6. Forehead exercise	My forehead is pleasantly cool. My facial muscles are relaxed.

Table 9: Classical AT Exercises

AT FOR ATHLETES

Learning Autogenic Training for sport is both different from and significantly shorter than Schultz's process in psychotherapy. In sports, AT is used to raise a healthy athlete's mental and physical performance to a higher level, and to increase his or her capacity for hard training. It is assumed that a healthy, physically trained athlete can learn to relax his or her muscles more easily and more quickly than patients in psychotherapy. Other assumptions about sport-modified AT are based on experience and on scientific studies on the use of AT for sports in eastern Europe.

For the athlete, the use of AT can have many benefits. AT helps the athlete to calm or activate his or her mental state and to change his or her thoughts, emotions, and self-confidence. AT can help athletes to recover more quickly during competition and practice. It can help athletes to relax more, so that they can maintain attention to the task at hand. It can also help athletes avoid undesirable thoughts, images, and habits. It can aid competitors in keeping an emotional balance and in activating or calming the proper emotions prior to or during competitions. AT can improve performance and eliminate the disturbing internal thoughts and feelings that often occur before important competitions. With AT, it is possible to learn enhancing new skills and techniques in a sport more rapidly and more easily than before.

When applying AT to sport, one must consider the specific, concrete demands of the sport and the particular problems of the athlete, as well as the athlete's own personal abilities. In other words, AT is both sport specific and individual specific.

LEARNING AUTOGENIC TRAINING

This section will teach athletes to induce the autogenic state rapidly and to control thoughts and emotions, even under unpleasant or stressful conditions. It will help athletes learn how to use their power and energy fully and how to create individual autogenic phrases and suggestions that are suited to particular competitive situations. The procedure, discussed in detail here, is summarized in Tables 10-12 on Pages 192 and 193.

Sport-modified AT takes 4 weeks of practice, 3 times daily, for 2 to 3 minutes. You will begin with preparation exercises, which help you to feel calm and relaxed. You will finish with activation exercises, which eliminate feelings of drowsiness and allow you to resume practice or competition with complete alertness.

Over the 4 weeks of initial training, you will gradually include more exercises and more parts of the body. During the first 2 weeks, you will do four autogenic exercises:

1. Encouraging feelings of heaviness (heaviness exercise)
2. Encouraging feelings of warmth (warmth exercise)
3. Encouraging feelings of calm and regular breathing (respiration exercise)
4. Encouraging feelings of a strong and quiet heartbeat (cardiac exercise)

These exercises will focus on both arms during the first week and both legs during the second week. During the third week and thereafter, you will practice two additional exercises:

5. Encouraging feelings of warmth in the solar plexus (solar plexus exercise)
6. Encouraging feelings of a cool forehead (forehead exercise)

In addition, focus attention on sensations of heaviness and warmth not just in the arms and legs but throughout the entire body as well.

WEEK ONE: EXERCISING BOTH ARMS

Choose a quiet, comfortable room in which to practice. Lie on your back (perhaps on a bed or sofa) and assume a comfortable position. You may put a pillow under your head. However, your neck must not have an unnatural bend or be in a stretched position. Place your arms down beside your body. As an alternative, you may practice these exercises in a sitting position.

PREPARATORY EXERCISES

Close your eyes and let yourself go. Take 3 deep comfortable breaths. Begin preparing for concentration. To prepare yourself for this state, you must be aware of your quiet tranquillity. Repeat in your mind, *"I am calm, totally calm."* Visualize this calmness in your mind. Concentrate on the image of calmness. Your concentration should be passive concentration rather than the active concentration normally required for reality-oriented tasks. Do not actually try to achieve this state. Instead of trying or striving, just let yourself go into this state.

Draw your attention away from action, either past or future. Be aware that you have sufficient time to practice and that you will totally relax. Allow your muscles to relax. Let all your muscles soften. Let them go limp. Slowly repeat in your mind the autogenic phrase, *"My whole body is relaxing."* Repeat it 2-3 times.

HEAVINESS EXERCISE

After experiencing relaxation, let yourself experience the sensation of heaviness.

Slowly repeat to yourself, *"My arms are relaxed."* Repeat it 2-3 times.

Then, repeat to yourself, *"My arms are heavy, very heavy."* Repeat it 3-4 times.

Focus your attention on your arms. Feel your arms relaxing and feeling heavier and heavier. Use your imagination to help induce the sensation of heaviness. Remember always to attend passively-without striving or trying. Let it happen.

Don't be discouraged if at first the sensation of heaviness is minor, or not felt at all. With practice, the feeling will appear and, over time, will become more pronounced

WARMTH EXERCISE

After practicing heaviness, now focus on feeling the sensation of warmth.

Slowly repeat to yourself 3-4 times, *"My arms are warm, very warm."* Focus your attention by "seeing" your arms and experiencing the sensation of warmth. Use your imagination to induce this feeling. For instance, visualize and feel the warmth of the sun on your skin, or the sensation of warmth in a hot tub or whirlpool or some other familiar source of warmth. Use passive concentration and let it happen.

The image and visualization of warmth is accompanied by relaxation of the arteries and capillaries. This means that they enlarge, allowing an increase in blood supply into those areas of the body upon which you are focusing-in this case, the arms. After learning this exercise you will not only have a feeling of warmth, but, as well, the areas where you focus will actually increase in temperature.

CALM BREATHING EXERCISE

After practicing the exercises above, move on to the respiration exercise. Concentrate on the autogenic phrases, *"My breath is calm and regular,"* and *"I am breathing easily."* Repeat them slowly 4-5 times. This exercise's goal is easy, regular breathing. Inhale by moving your stomach outward and exhale by moving your stomach inward. This quiet breathing will have a pleasant, calming effect on you. When the exercise is well executed, you will find yourself concentrating on your breathing as you perceive the regularity of your automatic breathing. You will be extremely aware of the quietness of your breath.

Anxiety and stress are commonly connected with respiratory irregularities. This exercise is helpful for eliminating the symptoms of stress, and thus for quieting the autonomic system.

CARDIAC (HEARTBEAT) EXERCISE

Following the respiratory exercise, you should then work on the cardiac exercise. However, I recommend that anyone suffering from a heart disorder of any kind should not engage in this exercise only after consultation with the doctor.

The goal of the cardiac exercise is to learn to feel the quiet beating of your heart. People are usually aware of their heartbeat only when under stress or in the midst of vigorous activity. This is when the heart is working its hardest. Most people, when they are resting quietly, do not consciously perceive the beating of their heart.

After recalling the sensations described above—relaxation, the sensation of heaviness, the sensation of warmth, and the sensation of calm breathing—you should concentrate on the phrase, *"My heartbeat is quiet and strong."* Repeat this phrase slowly, 5-6 times. This exercise sets in motion a sequence in which various elements stimulate each other: When your heart has a quiet rhythm, this increases your peace of mind. Peace of mind strengthens relaxation. In turn, relaxation strengthens the quietness of your heart rhythm.

You may find that putting your hand over the heart area during the exercise will facilitate heightened awareness of your heartbeat. It will disturb the feelings of relaxation in your arm, but it is only a temporarily maneuver.

ACTIVATION EXERCISES

An AT session always ends with three exercises to return you to the normal waking state: taking a deep breath, opening the eyes, and briskly moving the arms and legs. These exercises are executed as follows:

Give yourself (in order) these self-commands: *"Deep breath,"* *"Open the eyes,"* and *"Exercise with the arms."*

Next, repeat these self-suggestion statements to yourself: *"Strength is returning to my arms and legs,"* and *"I am feeling fresh and reenergized."*

Exercising the arms means stretching and flexing the arms, followed by energetic movements.

RULES, GUIDELINES FOR PRACTICING AT

- **Frequency of Practice**. Try to practice 3 times daily. If you can't, it is better to practice 2 times a day regularly than to try practicing 4 times a day occasionally.

- **Duration of Practice**. Practice should only last 2 to 3 minutes, even if the desired effects do not occur. Longer practice can be counterproductive, leading to increased tension.

- **Time of Practice**. Try to develop a daily practice rhythm. Pick a time of day that works best, and practice at that same time each day.

- **Position**. I suggest practicing AT in both lying and sitting positions. The desired effects often occur more quickly in a prone position. However, you may be forced at times to practice in a sitting position (for example, at a competition). Therefore, I suggest that you alternate between the lying and sitting positions when you practice. In both cases, the position must be comfortable so that the whole body is able to relax. In the lying position, the feet are slightly apart with the toes slightly turned out. The arms are beside the body, slightly bent at the elbows.

- The sitting position has several variations, depending primarily upon the chair. It can be more difficult to avoid muscle tension in a sitting position. Therefore, attention to the position is important. If possible, support your back comfortably against the chair. Legs are slightly apart, toes slightly turned out, and feet are flat on the floor. If the chair is too high and your feet do not touch the floor, put a pillow or blanket under the feet for support.

  If the chair has armrests, place your forearms on the supports with your hands hanging freely over the front of the rests. If the chair has no arm support, place your forearms on your thighs. Your arms should not be touching each other. Of course, your comfort is foremost, and if a variation in the above position is necessary, feel free to go ahead with it.

- **Termination of AT.** AT should always terminate with activation exercises, even during the times that the desired sensations do not occur.

- **Keep a Training Log**. I strongly recommend a systematic recording of all AT exercises. Keep track of the frequency of practice, progress occurring over time, specific sensations that occur each session, and manifestations that occur as a result of your practice, such as a general sense of well-being or improvement in your sport. This information is vital if you have the opportunity to consult with a specialist in AT. A sample of how to keep an AT training log can be found in Appendix B.

- **Transition to the Next Exercise**. General guidelines, provided in this chapter, describe the amount of time to spend on each exercise. An alternative guideline can be used to continue executing each exercise until the desired result has been obtained on two consecutive days. For some, this may occur either earlier or later than the suggested time limits.

- **When Not to Train.** In cases of illness, AT should not be practiced. Illness can disturb the practice and negatively influence the results.

- **Using a Tape Recorder.** I generally do not recommend using a tape recorder for learning the AT exercises. The phrases are short, and memorizing them offers the advantage of being able to practice anytime in any place. However, if you think that a tape recorder will be helpful, go ahead and tape yourself repeating the phrases slowly. When listening to the tape, concentrate fully on the suggestions.

- **Importance of Activation.** I cannot emphasize enough that each practice session of AT should finish with activation exercises. End each exercise session with these energetic inner commands: *"Deep breath,"* *"Open eyes,"* and *"Exercise the arms."* Then sit or stand up and make energetic movements with your arms to get rid of the heaviness. When practicing in bed before going to sleep, the relaxation need not be disturbed by this command.

- During competition and practice, you must quickly come back to an alert* state. This means ridding yourself of drowsiness and the sensation of heaviness. You need to learn to make the whole process automatic so that you can quickly get back to your best level and continue your performance. Also remember, however, to be patient—you must practice the procedures consistently, but without forcing them.

- **Progress Takes Time.** During AT you will experience a number of physical sensations: limb heaviness and warmth, warmth in the epigastric (stomach) region, a drowsy state, and sensations of heaviness or floating when you shift to a calm state (this is known as parasympathetic dominance). At first you may not see progress in inducing these sensations. Sometimes there is an increase in excitation and tension while learning the techniques. The positive effects of AT happen only after systematic practice and training. Gradually your progress will accelerate. Relaxation will become deeper, visualization will be clearer, and bodily sensations will become more calming.

- **The Process of Concentration in AT.** You can concentrate on autosuggestive phrases using two methods. You should learn and use both techniques. The first consists of mechanically repeating the autosuggestive phrase in your mind. The second method involves imagining or visualizing attributes of the desired state as fully as possible. For instance, if you are attempting a heaviness exercise, you could imagine the qualities of heaviness with as much vividness as you can. Imagine the effort it takes to move a heavy tree limb. Imagine the limb pressing down on the couch or floor you're lying on. Picture its magnitude and weightiness.

Practical AT Guidelines

In the application of AT to sports, the following guidelines enhance the overall effectiveness of the regimen.

- Attention should be passively focused on the specific part of the body, and the autosuggestive phrases should be spoken internally as that part of the body is visualized.

- Autosuggestive phrases should be repeated slowly several times, allowing time for awareness of the autosuggestion to register. The autosuggestions are interspersed with visual imagery. For example, the athlete can focus attention on the arms, visualizing them completely relaxed, resting on the floor, dissociated from his or her body, limp and relaxed with a feeling of induced heaviness.

- Prior experiences or memories ("helping" images) can be used to heighten the effect. For example, you can imagine the feeling of the warmth of the sun on your skin, or of a hot bath, or the feeling of a cool breeze or touch on your forehead.

- No conscious effort should be made to deepen or control breathing during the respiration exercise. The athlete should direct his or her attention to the nature, even rhythm of the diaphragm. Breathing is natural and completely automatic. In all cases the athlete merely repeats the autosuggestive phrase(s) and passively experiences the sensation that follows.

Week Two: Exercising Both Legs

Calmness

Start each AT session with the preparation exercises used during the first week, beginning with, "*I am totally calm*" and "*My whole body is relaxed.*"

HEAVINESS EXERCISE

First, induce the learned sensation of heaviness in your arms. Next, let yourself experience the sensation of heaviness in your legs.

Slowly repeat to yourself, *"My legs are relaxed."* Say it 2-3 times.

Then say, *"My legs are heavy, very heavy."* Say this 3-5 times. Again, use your imagination vividly to help to induce the sensation of heaviness.

Focus your attention by visualizing your legs. Feel the heaviness happen, visualize it happening, and let it happen. Remember always to attend passively—without striving or trying.

WARMTH EXERCISE

After practicing heaviness, let yourself experience the sensation of warmth.

First, induce the learned sensation of warmth in your arms and legs. Then focus your attention on your legs.

Slowly say to yourself two to three times, *"My legs are warm, very warm."* As before, focus your attention by losing your legs and experiencing the sensation of warmth in your legs. Feel the warmth move from your thighs down toward your knee, calf, foot, and toes. Again, use a vivid image to visualize warmth.

CALM BREATHING EXERCISE

As during the first week, allow yourself to experience the sensation of calm, regular breathing. Use a phrase such as, *"My breath is calm and regular."* Use the same instructions as for week one.

CARDIAC (HEARTBEAT) EXERCISE

Use the same procedure as you did during the first week to experience a strong, quiet heartbeat.

Silently say this 5-6 times: *"My heartbeat is strong and quiet."*

ACTIVATION EXERCISES

As during the first week, conclude the exercise session with these phrases: *"Open eyes." "Deep breath." "Exercise the arms and legs." "Strength is returning to my arms and legs." "I am feeling fresh and reenergized."*

WEEK THREE: EXERCISING THE WHOLE BODY

CALMNESS

Use the same preparation exercises as those used during the first two weeks. Begin with these statements: *"I am totally calm." "My whole body is relaxing."*

HEAVINESS

Repeat 4-5 times, *"Both arms and legs are heavy,"* followed by, *"The whole body is heavy."* While repeating these statements, visualize and imagine heaviness as perfectly and as vividly as you can.

WARMTH

Repeat 4-5 times, *"Both arms and legs are warm,"* and then, *"The whole body is warm."* Again, use the phrases and visualize warmth as perfectly as possible.

CALM BREATHING

Use the same procedure as during the first two weeks.

CARDIAC (HEARTBEAT) EXERCISE

Use the same procedure as during the first two weeks.

SOLAR PLEXUS WARMTH

Focus your attention on your solar plexus (just below the rib cage). Let yourself experience a feeling of warmth in your solar plexus, perhaps by imagining warm sunlight pouring onto your stomach. Feel the warmth, and let it happen.

Say slowly to yourself, four to five times, *"Warmth is pouring into the solar plexus. My solar plexus is warm."*

In your mind, see the warmth spreading from the chest gradually down, warming the whole area, both from within and from without.

The goal of the solar plexus exercise is to calm and regularize the functioning of the organs in your stomach cavity. It can be very helpful in decreasing your anxiety and can create a pleasant, relaxed, tranquil state.

THE COOL FOREHEAD EXERCISE

Next focus your attention on your face and forehead.

See your forehead, and slowly say, 5-6 times, *"My facial muscles are relaxed,"* and then, *"My forehead is pleasantly cool."*

Imagine a pleasantly cool sensation on your forehead, perhaps a gentle wind.

WEEK FOUR: MASTERING THE SKILLS

During the first 3 weeks you were exposed to all the basic AT exercises. In week four you want to become entirely comfortable practicing them. This section includes several techniques for individualizing the process. Table 9-12 contain the phrases learned during the first 3 weeks. Use them to help you memorize the phrases. Once you have done so, you may want to shorten the AT phrases. Finally, the Ericksonian approach is offered as an alternative method of practicing AT.

Athletes who seek to learn AT must practice regularly and systematically. They must literally follow a training schedule. A blank protocol for practicing Autogenic Training is provided in Appendix B.

At the end of week four you should have a short, concise methodology to quickly get into a state of deep relaxation and heightened concentration.

Research in sports has shown that short, frequent practice sessions are more effective than long, protracted practice—especially if there are long breaks between practice sessions. Thus, the best way to learn AT is as suggested: 3 times daily, for 2 to 3 minutes each time.

After mastering the basic form of AT, it is possible to use a shortened form of the phrases. Sometimes the phrases can be shortened to three or four words, resulting in more intense images. Examples of this are:

"Totally calm." "Totally relaxed." "My body is very heavy." "The warmth is increasing in my body." "Cool forehead." "Clear thoughts." The self-suggestion phrases help to activate mind and body, and are an important part of AT. It is, therefore, important to practice these phrases.

After a couple of weeks, you can systematically eliminate any external help, such as verbal instruction or tape recordings. In this way, you learn to rely on yourself, rather than maintaining a dependency on external assistance. Once these exercises have been mastered, AT can be used in real situations involving training and competition.

Using an Ericksonian Approach to AT

The late Milton Erickson, M.D., used hypnotic suggestion in an unusual way. As you learn the basic steps of AT, you can take advantage of his Utilization Approach, which is explained further in Appendix A. It involves being aware of your own unique sensations and experiences, and slightly modifying the basic autogenic exercises.

For example, one of my students always experienced a pleasant numbness in his limbs when practicing the heaviness exercise. He then changed the autogenic statement for this exercise to, "My arms and legs are pleasantly numb," rather than, "My arms are heavy."

Another of my students, who experienced lightness of his limbs and body instead of heaviness, used the autogenic phrases, "My body is light, very light," and "Like floating in the air."

One of my students, a world-class U.S. rower, changed the order of the autogenic exercises. He finds it is more effective to start with the respiratory exercise, so he practices that first and then goes on to the heaviness exercises.

Some athletes are able to work on the whole body almost from the start of AT. They are able, almost immediately, to experience sensations of heaviness, warmth, and so on throughout the entire body. Some have practiced all six of the autogenic exercises from the first or second week. Their experience and observations have proven the effectiveness of this method.

I am not suggesting that you skip some steps in learning the basic AT. Most of my athletes have successfully followed the steps that you have just read about. However, I encourage you, as I have with my own athletes, to use your own unique, ongoing experience to develop the autogenic state. This is the essence of Erickson's utilization approach.

Week 1: Exercising Both Arms	
Preparation	I am totally calm. My whole body is relaxing.
Heaviness	My arms are relaxed. Both arms are heavy, very heavy.
Warmth	My arms are warm, very warm.
Respiration	My breath is quiet and regular.
Cardiac	My heart beat is strong and quiet.
Activation	Deep breath and open the eyes.
	Exercise the arms.
	The feelings of heaviness are eliminated.
	Strength is returning to my arms and legs.
	I am feeling fresh and reenergized.

Table 10: Exercising Both Arms

Week 2: Exercising Both Legs	
Preparation	I am totally calm. My whole body is relaxing.
Heaviness	My legs are relaxed. Both legs are heavy, very heavy.
Warmth	My legs are warm, very warm.
Respiration	My breath is quiet and regular.
Cardiac	My heartbeat is strong and quiet.
Activation	Deep breath and open the eyes. Exercise the legs. The feelings of heaviness are eliminated. Strength is returning to my arms and legs. I am feeling fresh and reenergized.

Table 11: Exercising Both Legs

Week 3: Exercising the Whole Body

Preparation	I am totally calm. My whole body is relaxing.
Heaviness	My arms and legs are relaxed. My arms and legs are heavy, very heavy. The whole body is heavy.
Warmth	My arms and legs are warm, very warm.
Respiratory	My breath is quiet and regular.
Cardiac	My heart beat is strong and quiet.
Solar Plexus	My solar plexus (stomach) is very warm. Warmth is pouring into the solar plexus.
Forehead	My facial muscles are relaxed and my forehead is pleasantly cool.
Activation	Deep breath. Open the eyes. Exercise the arms and legs. The whole body is refreshed. The feelings of heaviness are eliminated. Strength is returning to my arms and legs. I am feeling fresh and reenergized.

Table 12: Exercising the Whole Body

15

INDIVIDUALLY TAILORED AUTOGENIC TRAINING

Sport-modified AT has a strong foundation in research. Literally thousands of athletes in eastern and western Europe use it as their "bible" in mental preparation. Once an athlete has learned basic AT, he or she can tailor it to his or her specific sport and situation. Here's how it works.

In basic AT, the heightened autogenic state (altered state) itself has a positive effect. You can utilize it for mind/body relaxation, for decreasing a high level of arousal and tension, and as an anti-stress device. The autogenic state is also a vehicle for applying individual-specific autogenic phrases as well as other mental techniques.

In summary, mastering basic AT takes 4 weeks, 3 times daily, for 2 to 3 minutes at a time. AT creates a heightened state of awareness (altered state) in which the athlete is receptive to suggestions and images. After learning basic AT, you can use this heightened state as a vehicle for applying the created individual-specific autogenic phrases to fit your own needs. In competition, athletes use the positive phrases and images that were rehearsed in practice to counter any negative thoughts or feelings that may arise during competition.

DESIGNING INDIVIDUALLY TAILORED AT

The individual-specific autogenic phrases are similar to posthypnotic suggestions. When creating individual-specific autogenic phrases, motivation has a significant role. The phrases should express certain needs and desires of the athlete. First, the athlete must desire a change. This desire will in turn determine the content of the phrases.

According to Schultz, an ideal case is when a person in a state of deep relaxation—a heightened state—experiences the individual/specific autogenic phrases so intensively that later, at a given time, they will occur totally automatically without any voluntary effort. Studies with posthypnotic suggestions show that such an effect can be achieved by training.

Schultz's student, Thomas, has suggested that individualized autogenic phrases should be short, positive, rhythmic, and clear, and should suggest specific action. The phrases must have meaning for the individual Short suggestive phrases have a better chance for success than long ones that contain too many details. Thomas also pointed out that, as in the case with any rules, sometimes exceptions are necessary to meet a specific individual's needs.

I agree with Thomas's assessment. I also suggest that the athlete write out the proposed phrases, and then, in order to gain clarity, discuss them with someone familiar with the AT process.

The student should then practice the phrases, using a technique similar to the one used when practicing the basic autogenic exercises (see Chapter 16). This means that the athlete should first repeat the phrase to himself or herself and then visualize himself or herself behaving in accordance with the suggestion. The image should be as clear and precise as possible.

In sport, individualized AT phrases are often used for two main purposes:

- To help the athlete withstand the rigors of the intensive, hard training (often referred to as the training load). Staying focused on hard training can be difficult, and is often accompanied by unpleasant emotions. Keeping your resolve to work hard can also be difficult in the face of distractions. AT phrases can be developed to help increase your resolve and make the training process more enjoyable. Typical phrases can include, "*I enjoy hard training,*" "*Training hard will permanently improve my performance,*" and "*I can withstand hard training.*"

- To strengthen self-confidence and self-assurance throughout the competition. Examples of such phrases are, "*I am totally calm and full of energy and strength during the competition,"* and *"I am always able to produce my best performance when I need to."*

The phrases should be individualized. Athletes must use their own words. It is quite typical for two athletes with the same goals to create entirely different phrases to accomplish the desired result.

STEP 1: CONCENTRATIVE ANALYSIS

Over the years, from observation of and conversations with my fencers, I have noticed big differences between their best and worst bouts. The differences are evident in all parts of the experience, including level of arousal, concentration, self-confidence, stress, self-talk, and muscle tension. To better study and understand these phenomena, I developed a method that I call concentrative analysis. With one of my fencers I induced a light hypnotic trance state and asked him to recall as vividly as he could all the details of his best competitive bout. I gave him questions like:

- What was the level of your arousal (on a scale of 0 to 10)? What was the level of your concentration (on a scale of 0 to 10)?
- What was the level of your self-confidence (on a scale of 0 to 10)?
- What was the level of your concern (stress) about performing well (on a scale of 0 to 10)?
- What was the level of nervousness (on a scale of 0 to 10)?
- What was the level of tension in different muscle groups (on a scale of 0 to 10)?
- What self-talk (inner monologue) did you have?
- What images and thoughts did you have?
- What did you picture?
- How and what did you see and hear?
- What was your emotional state and your physiological state?

I recorded all his vivid, sensory, detailed answers on a tape recorder. I then asked the same questions about his worst competitive bout.

I took the information and compared his best and worst bouts. The comparisons helped me to recognize what was stopping him from achieving greater success. One thing that stood out was that his self-talk when fencing his best consisted of short, positive, motivational, and suggestive phrases. The positive self-talk was an excellent place to begin when looking for individualized autogenic phrases.

I have found over the years that this technique can help me identify my athletes' problems. The types of issues that will limit progression often include lack of self-confidence, excessive arousal, extreme muscle tension in specified areas, fear of competing against certain opponents, or errors in technique or tactics.

As I mentioned before, the concentrative analysis revealed self-talk became the basis for individualized autogenic phrases. Phrases designed this way are effective because they are spontaneously created by the athletes themselves. In this case they mirrored the athletes' own self-talk in that they were short, motivational, and suggestive. The athletes liked them because they were easy to remember. In addition, the phrases were taken from the best performances; therefore, the self-talk was already associated with success.

Most athletes who did concentrative analyses were surprised by what they discovered. They realized that they had been unaware of their inner monologue and sensory perceptions.

LEARNING CONCENTRATIVE ANALYSIS

The first step in designing individualized phrases uses concentrative analysis. As mentioned above, this analysis involves visualizing your best and worst performances in great and vivid detail.

Before attempting concentrative analysis, first learn the basic autogenic techniques described in Chapter 14. When you are ready to do the analysis, sit or lie down in a comfortable position. Close your eyes and induce the autogenic state. Then recall your best and later your worst bout or competition. Record in your training diary everything you remember, vividly and in great detail. The charts that follow and the concentrative

CONCENTRATIVE ANALYSIS WORKSHEET
BEST PERFORMANCE

Instructions: In either a sitting or reclining position close your eyes and bring on the autogenic state. Recall as vividly as possible everything you can about your very best performance. To stimulate your timing, ask yourself the following 10 questions about your best performance. The answers to these questions may vary greatly from athlete to athlete. When you are finished, record as much detail as you can.

Arousal level	0	1	2	3	4	5	6	7	8	9	10
Level of concern about performance	0	1	2	3	4	5	6	7	8	9	10
Level of Nervousness	0	1	2	3	4	5	6	7	8	9	10
Concentration level	0	1	2	3	4	5	6	7	8	9	10
Confidence level	0	1	2	3	4	5	6	7	8	9	10

Amount of muscle tension

legs	0	1	2	3	4	5	6	7	8	9	10
arms, shoulders	0	1	2	3	4	5	6	7	8	9	10
face, neck	0	1	2	3	4	5	6	7	8	9	10

Images, visualizations

What I saw and heard around me

Self-talk

Emotional state

Physiological state

Table 13: Concentrative Analysis Worksheet Best Performance

CONCENTRATIVE ANALYSIS WORKSHEET
WORST PERFORMANCE

Instructions: In either a sitting or reclining position close your eyes and bring on the autogenic state. Recall as vividly as possible everything you can about your very best performance. To stimulate your timing, ask yourself the following 10 questions about your best performance. The answers to these questions may vary greatly from athlete to athlete. When you are finished, record as much detail as you can.

Arousal level	0	1	2	3	4	5	6	7	8	9	10
Level of concern about performance	0	1	2	3	4	5	6	7	8	9	10
Level of Nervousness	0	1	2	3	4	5	6	7	8	9	10
Concentration level	0	1	2	3	4	5	6	7	8	9	10
Confidence level	0	1	2	3	4	5	6	7	8	9	10

Amount of muscle tension

legs	0	1	2	3	4	5	6	7	8	9	10
arms, shoulders	0	1	2	3	4	5	6	7	8	9	10
face, neck	0	1	2	3	4	5	6	7	8	9	10

Images, visualizations

What I saw and heard around me

Self-talk

Emotional state

Physiological state

Table 14: Concentrative Analysis Worksheet Worst Performance

analyses of top athletes in Chapter 16 will help you. The analysis is extremely important since it is the primary source for creating individual-specific autogenic phrases.

If you find this exercise difficult, the following examples may help you get started. However, be sure when you are performing concentrative analysis that you are describing your own experience. You must use words that make sense to you.

ATHLETE'S BEST PERFORMANCES

What I saw when I performed at my best:
- The fencing strip, my opponent, the director, the weapon, my coach.
- The lines in the bottom of the swimming pool, the spectators.

What I visualized or imagined when I performed at my best:
- I saw myself attacking my opponent.
- I had the image of anticipating my opponent's responses.
- I had the image of... (doing a particular movement).

What I heard:
- The sound of the fencing blades.
- The sound of the ball against the racquet.
- The sound of my foot movement, my breathing.
- Cheering; my opponent's cry when she won a point; background noise.

What self-talk or self-suggestions I had:
- Stay loose; do not rush; concentrate; one move at a time; focus; stay low.

What I felt physically:
- Tension in my shoulder (or other muscle groups).
- Sweating.
- A tingling sensation.
- A knot in my stomach.
- Awareness of my own breathing or heartbeat.

What my emotional state was:

- I felt loose, relaxed, alert, focused, confident, afraid, angry, and happy. Others might say, "In the zone."—totally focused.

The answers to these questions vary greatly from athlete to athlete. Describe your internal and external sensations—your mood, emotions, thoughts, and images—and the self-talk you experienced.

After analyzing your best, most successful performance, you should do a concentrative analysis on your worst, most unsuccessful performance. The reason for doing so is to identify how your mind works when doing your best and worst.

A very effective method of concentrative analysis is watching your most successful performance from a videotape. Sit comfortably, relax, and induce the autogenic state. Then turn on the VCR and watch your best performance. Recall all your feelings, thoughts, images, self-talk, and levels of arousal, concentration, self-confidence, and so on. Do not evaluate your actions or technique. Focus only on the emotions, feelings, and images you had in a very detailed and vivid way. Then write it down in your diary.

Do the same watching your worst performance. Compare the differences in detail. Now repeat the exercise, but this time, approach your performance from the aspect of technique and tactics. Also, notice the accompanying feelings, thoughts, and self-talk.

After concentrative analyses of their best and worst performances, athletes report surprise about how differently they talk to themselves, see, feel, and think during their best performance as compared with their worst.

STEP 2: CREATING PHRASES

Based on the concentrative analysis in Step 1, identify what is stopping you from improving. What was the difference between your best and your worst performances?

The autogenic phrases that you construct will serve as cues to bring on positive feelings and will turn negative thoughts and self-talk into positive ones. The phrases will trigger self-confidence, relaxed but focused alertness, and the feelings of victory that have accompanied your very best performance. They will also help you to correct bad habits.

Follow this methodology when designing phrases:

- Make the most of the positive self-talk, thoughts, images, and feelings that you have experienced during your best performance.

- Also focus on your negative self-talk and thoughts from poor performances. Change them to positive self-talk as a step toward eliminating negative habits and problems.

- Record in your training diary the specific autogenic phrases that you wish to use.

The real-life examples that follow will help you better understand the process of creating individual-specific autogenic phrases.

One of my saber fencers had serious problems, becoming very angry, upset, and distracted by what he considered to be bad calls by the referee. I suggested that he use these autogenic phrases: "*I am totally indifferent to the director's calls,*" and "*I am relaxed, calm, and focused.*" He practiced daily, seeing himself as relaxed, calm, focused, and indifferent to the director's calls while repeating his autogenic phrases.

In addition, I suggested that he visualize a fencer whom he considered a role model and imagine how that fencer would react in similar circumstances. My student practiced daily. After two weeks he was able to eliminate his problem.

A cross-country skier's concentrative analysis indicated that he had a specific problem at certain point on the track. When going uphill, he felt tired to the point of exhaustion and experienced both pain and negative thoughts that he could not race uphill. The following autogenic phrases were created to help him to overcome his difficulties:

- I imagine and feel a rope that is connected to my center of gravity and is pulling me along.
- I am pulled with more and more force along the way.
- I imagine and feel a very strong wind pushing me forward.
- My strides are now easier and faster.

- I imagine and feel my teammate pushing me forward with great strength.

Many times the athlete's positive self-talk, thoughts, and self-commands of his or her best performance are used as autogenic phrases or as cues for recreating a similar feeling or mood or eliminating the negative self-talk. Those cues can be used deliberately.

Notice in the concentrative analyses that follow in Chapter 16 that the suggested autogenic phrases use the athlete's own self-talk-the same things he or she says unconsciously when performing his or her best.

I suggest doing this since I view the athlete's positive self-talk as a "computer program" stored in the subconscious that is used spontaneously and unconsciously for affirmation—strengthening the athlete's confidence, belief, and attitude. In addition, this self-talk seems to serve the purpose of a "race plan"—spontaneous, brief instructions during different phases of the performance that help the athlete focus on the task at hand.

In addition, athletes' self-talk when performing their best provides them with short commands to focus-for example on an external object or internal body process. This helps them to eliminate any distractions or negative thoughts and keep their minds from wandering to the past or future. When performing their best athletes always focused on the present and this was reflected in their self-talk. On the other hand, when performing their worst athletes tend to focus on the past or future. They worry and ruminate, and the context of their self-talk consists of their stored negative problems and learned limitations.

From my observations athletes on their own have the natural capability to manage themselves successfully. From reviewing their self-talk when performing their best, it is clear that they spontaneously give themselves positive affirmations, instruct themselves to stay focused, and naturally develop "race plans"—to help control their minds. Therefore, the individually-tailored autogenic phrases can be based on the "blueprint" of an athletes' positive self-talk when performing his or her best. This helps the athlete to bring his or her subconscious affirmations, self-strengthening commands, and reinforcing instructions into conscious awareness, allowing the athlete access to these thoughts more freely and more often.

On the other hand, individualized phrases sometimes are used to overcome problems that the athlete is not able to cope with on his or her own. For example, the athlete's concentrative analysis could identify a lack of confidence, lack of concentration, errors in tactics and techniques, and so on. For example, one of my fencers, temporarily on a losing streak, lost his self-belief and his confidence in his own ability to achieve victory. I suggested that he use these autogenic phrases: *"I trained very hard and well." "I have beaten many top world-class fencers in the past." "I believe in myself."* In addition, I suggested that he watch his most successful bouts from the World Cups and World Championships on videotape on a daily basis during the week before his competition. He soon regained his confidence and self-belief.

I suggest that you carefully study the examples of concentrative analyses that appear in Chapter 14. Notice the differences in sensations, self-talk, imagery, moods, and so on between the best and worst performances. Also take note of the suggested individual autogenic phrases. Through this careful attention you will gain an understanding of the concentrative analysis process. This will help you to develop your own individual-specific autogenic phrases.

STEP 3: RULES FOR DESIGNING AUTOGENIC PHRASES

In order to successfully eliminate bad habits, you must follow certain guidelines in creating individualized autogenic phrases. The following list will help.

1. The phrases must always be positive. Never mention the negative ideas, because what is expected tends to happen.

2. Always use the present tense. Imagine that what you are suggesting is true not sometime in the future, but now.

3. Use only one phrase at a time. Using many suggestions in the same sentence weakens the effect of them all. Choose one main suggestion and work on it until you have absorbed it.

4. Make your phrases short, clear, and simple. Use words that a 10-year-old would understand. Do not use long, complex sentences.

5. Imagine yourself carrying out the phrases. For instance if you suffer from stage fright, use the phrase, "*I am quiet and relaxed when performing,*" or "*I am quiet and brave in front of spectators.*" See yourself standing calmly and confidently before the crowd.

6. Use the formulas in connection with concrete situations. As you apply the formula to yourself, imagine yourself in the competition setting.

7. Newly constructed phrases should allow you to use your imagination to visualize yourself carrying out the individualized phrases.

8. Your suggestions should always be in words that are natural to you. If the words do not come naturally, they will not seem to apply to you.

Step 4: Anchoring

My athletes practice anchoring, or associating their positive feelings with a physical cue when they practice AT. They induce the desired positive emotions—feelings of confidence, strength, determination, and so on—and then press the thumb to the index finger while recalling the images associated with the positive emotions. The movement of pressing thumb to index finger is just like holding the weapon during a fencing bout. This motion helps the fencer connect with the sport and focus on the power of the positive emotion it evokes.

During competition, the fencers use this same tiny movement, along with the individual autogenic phrases, whenever they start the bout, and whenever needed. The anchor and the phrases now trigger a conditioned response—an association with that winning feeling that helps them achieve their goals.

Anchoring involves recalling the experience of positive feelings of success, and then associating these feelings with touching the body or sport equipment.

STEP 5: DAILY PRACTICE

You should practice your specific, individualized autogenic phrases on a daily basis until you achieve your goal of improvement. Then go back to the phrases a day or two before the tournament for a tune-up. When you practice, do so as follows:

- Induce the autogenic state. Repeat your individual phases.
- See yourself behaving in the way that you want to.
- Recall or reexperience your positive feelings from your best performances, with the help of autogenic phrases.
- Anchor your positive feelings, for example, by pressing your thumb against your index finger as you do when you hold your weapon, while you experience these feelings.

The anchor and the autogenic phrases will be the cues for you during competition or training, available whenever you need to trigger the winning feelings of confidence, determination, and so forth.

PHRASES FOR PARTICULAR SITUATIONS

Many individualized phrases were developed for athletes to use during particular situations. Although phrases should be designed for the individual athlete through concentrative analysis (self-study), you may find the examples contained in the following sections and in the appendices helpful.

Because these samples are rather lengthy, the athlete may want to use a tape recorder as an aid in practicing them.

COPING WITH STRESS AND TENSION DURING COMPETITION

Competition creates a great deal of stress and tension in the athlete. Because the motor centers of the brain are in a state of increased stimulation, the athlete may become fatigued. This may negatively influence performance. In this case, AT can be used to reduce the state of tension and high arousal, and to speed up the process of regeneration (recovery). AT also helps to develop and maintain the optimal level of arousal necessary for competition. During competition, the competitor, when off the playfield can utilize the short or long breaks for the above-mentioned purposes.

Perfect mastery of AT has made it possible for top eastern European athletes to induce deep relaxation and to regenerate, even during a short pause in competition. Fencers, wrestlers, karate competitors, and other athletes often use AT during the pauses between bouts. Top boxers can induce an autogenic state for 30 seconds, during which they are more receptive to the coach's instructions. During the next 30 seconds, they are able to activate themselves. In this way, they can use a 60-second break to their utmost advantage.

Remember, in addition to decreasing the athlete's "over arousal," AT can be used when the athlete lacks energy or aggressiveness. Specific activating autogenic phrases and the intensive activation exercises are used for this purpose.

RAPID SWITCH-OFF AND RAPID RECOVERY

An example of AT phrases used during brief breaks in competition is presented below. It was prepared for two fencers, one a World Champion and the other a silver medalist in the World Championships. Both individuals used these phrases for intensive rest and fast recovery between bouts.

- I am completely relaxed.
- My whole body is resting and I feel refreshed.
- My breath is quiet and regular. (Repeat 2 to 4 times.)
- Also my heart is beating quietly, more quietly all the time.
- Both my arms are relaxed.
- Pleasant feelings of warmth are pouring into my body.
- The muscles in my face are relaxed.
- The muscles in my forehead, eyebrows, and lips are relaxed.
- Tension has been released.

- I feel quiet; my whole body is refreshed.
- My breath is quiet. After a few deep breaths, the feeling of heaviness is disappearing.
- I feel fresh and light.
- Strength is returning to my legs and arms.
- Deep breath.
- Open the eyes.
- Exercise the arms.

REJUVENATING THE ATHLETE

Athletes competing at the Moscow Olympics in fencing and modern pentathlon used the following autogenic phrases during breaks in training and competition.

- I am totally relaxed.
- My whole body is resting and I feel refreshed.
- My breath is calm and regular.
- I am totally relaxed.
- My whole body is resting and I feel refreshed.
- My breath is calm and regular.
- Also my heart is beating calmly, more quietly all the time.
- Both arms are relaxed.
- Pleasant feelings of warmth are pouring into my body.
- The muscles in my face are relaxed.
- The muscles in my forehead, eyebrows, and lips are relaxed.
- Tension has been released.
- I feel calm.
- My whole body is refreshed.
- My breath is calm.

- After a few deep breaths, the feeling of heaviness is disappearing.
- I feel fresh and light.
- Strength is returning to my legs and arms.
- Deep breath.
- Open eyes.
- Exercise the arms.

Again, it should again be emphasized that self-suggestive phrases are accompanied by the athlete's mental imagery. When you do the AT exercises, focus on the phrases or images without trying to rush or force them.

SUMMARY

Once you have practiced the basic AT exercises presented in Chapter 14 you are ready to develop your own individualized autogenic phrases to overcome particular concerns or problems. Individual-specific autogenic phrases are constructed through self-study, or concentrative analysis. After constructing appropriate phrases, practice them daily. During competition, use the individualized phrases and anchoring as ways to trigger feelings of confidence and to focus. When you master AT, you will be well on your way to self-regulation.

16

CONCENTRATIVE ANALYSIS OF OLYMPIC ATHLETES

The previous chapter described how to develop appropriate individualized autogenic phrases. Developing the phrases begins with a detailed concentrative analysis of the athlete's best and worst performances. In order to more fully understand the process, this chapter contains examples of the concentrative analyses of U.S. Olympic athletes. Following each example is the suggested autogenic phrases for each particular athlete.

The examples are interesting in and of themselves. They take you inside the minds of four successful athletes. Note the very detail that each athlete provides. The detail helps the athletes to more fully understand themselves and provides the basis for the autogenic phrases.

Although each of these athletes has agreed to have their names appear in this book, I have decided to keep their identities confidential to protect their privacy. I greatly appreciate their allowing me to share their fine work with you.

CONCENTRATIVE ANALYSIS OF OLYMPIC FENCER

PERFORMING HIS BEST

This fencer recorded the following information describing how he experienced his best performance. I know this fencer to be a very strong-willed and confident performer.

> I am charged up, anxious; I'm ready to go. I see my opponent as an adversary who is in my way. I want to go to the next

level. I see him as an obstacle. I want to push him aside, get him out of my way.

I am confident and focused, with a level of concentration of 9 on a scale of 0 to 10. My level of arousal is high, 8 to 9 on a scale of 0 to 10. I feel intense but relaxed. I feel in control.

My body is relaxed and warm. Sometimes I feel a few aches in my knees, but they quickly go away as soon as the bout begins. I feel sweat rolling down my face (as a result of warming up). Before starting the bout, I am a little nervous, but not overly anxious. I am wondering who I will fence. I am anxiously awaiting being called to the strip. I go over; who is my opponent? But I do not feel uptight. I smile and talk to people. I am anxious to start the bout.

When the name of my opponent is announced, and he is a top-level fencer, I feel a little nervous. I immediately think, *"Oh boy, it will be tough!"* Then I settle down and say to myself *"I can beat that person."* First I recall the coach saying that I can beat anybody out there if I do what I have been taught to do and have practiced. I feel that I have been practicing, working every day—taking lessons and/or doing free fencing. I reflect on that, and tell myself that I have been practicing, that I have beaten very strong fencers before, and that I can beat this one also. I get charged up and ready to go, but first I say, *"This is going to be a tough one to win—but I have the ability to do it,"* and then I relax and settle into the bout. I again feel that he is in my way and that I have to beat this person to go to the next level.

When a weaker fencer is announced as my opponent, I feel that I could and should beat this person. All I have to do is what I have been taught. I just have to settle down and not do stupid things and the bout should work out for me. I am not sure what I will do against this fencer, but I feel that the proper actions will come out of me during the bout. I can fence and beat him. I see the bout as time I have to put in to get to a higher level. I felt very confident that I will get the touch, and I do not worry about how long the bout takes. My arousal level is high. It is a very businesslike mood but I also think about mistakes that I've sometimes made, and I make sure not to take the bout for granted I make sure not to make mistakes, not to get tense, and to avoid being "uncharged" (flat).

When they announce the name of an unknown opponent, I wonder who this fencer is and what country he is from. Then l try to figure out how good a fencer he is by identifying the country he is from. But I realize that it does not matter how good a fencer he is, or how good his country is at fencing, because I have beaten people from the best fencing countries before, so I can beat this person also. I feel confident about the bout coming up and about what I will do against him then. But again, I try to recall and focus on my training and what I have been taught.

When the bout starts, I see only the image of the opponent. I see the outline of the fencer. I focus more on the image of the fencer before me. I see the outline of the opponent. I do not see him. I do not see his arms, head, and legs. I see his outline and I do not focus on him individually. I see his image—the overall picture. I can see the target area, the jacket, and with my peripheral vision, I see his saber.

I do not see the crowd. I do not see the director or the face of the opponent. I am aware of the distance of the strip behind me, where I am, where he (the opponent) is, and how much space he and I have. I see the outline of the opponent's upper body. I see the coach or Pete (teammate), but nobody else. I know exactly what I am doing. I am eager to try the next thing. I am in full control. Everything is concentrated on the opponent. I am completely in the bout—the strip, the opponent, and me. I am confident and I try and do more things, different actions using a larger repertoire.

Before I begin to fence, I picture the actions that I would like to take. I see myself doing the entire action (movement), or, sometimes, just the beginning of the action. I see myself as if on a TV screen. I have a general idea what to do in the whole bout, and I picture it. I am playing with different ideas (and see them in my head). For example, this fencer is an aggressive fencer, so maybe I should take the attack away from him. He likes to attack so I am going to attack first; (or) he likes to play defensively, so I am trying to draw him out and make him attack. I have these general ideas.

Maybe sometimes, late in the bout, I start considering what has gone on earlier. I may think, "*I am doing too many stop cuts. Do them, but not too often. Be careful, or he might figure it out!*" I wonder what he (opponent) is thinking of me. But I am in command—I am the commander, the dictator. Even if I retreat, I want to control the game, keeping my mind clear. I say to myself things like, "*Stay low; get down—I'm getting down deep; get low; I'm digging in the trenches; get low like a cat, like a tiger; stay loose; concentrate; hand low, and relaxed.*" Not only do I say these things to myself—I also picture myself doing them. I also say to myself, "*Think only about this touch.*"

PERFORMING HIS WORST

This athlete also learned a great deal about himself by doing a concentrative analysis in which he envisioned his worst performance. This information helps the athlete and the coach to formulate a strategy for improvement. The ultimate goal is to get the athlete to associate more strongly with the thoughts and feelings attached to his or her best performance.

My concentration is poor. I think more about the person rather than fencing the person. I have negative thoughts. I do not want to be on the strip. My confidence is low. I feel anxious, tight, and mentally tense. I picture myself getting hit. I also picture other images, not related to fencing—like what I did yesterday, what I will do tomorrow, other sports, and people playing other sports. I do not see myself doing the (proper) actions. I feel anxious and tight. I feel a little ache in my lower left back. I do not feel very warm. I feel a little tight in my shoulders and legs—like I'm stiff.

I felt very uncomfortable on the strip, like I am out of place. I feel very low in intensity, and I feel low arousal. My confidence is low. I think about so many things. This person can beat me! I feel the sensation of getting hit before my opponent touches me with the weapon. I see everything around me: the crowd, the director, people around the strip, and lots of people. I see my opponent's face, his family members, and his friends. I see the person instead of the image. I see all my teammates and family members.

I try to tell myself to get into the bout and to start fencing, or to do something. I think I am going to lose. I also say to myself, *"Oh, brother. You're going to lose the bout, but maybe you can get lucky and get a touch somehow."* I tell myself to try something else or I criticize myself all during the bout. I also tell myself *"Try—maybe you'll get lucky."* I hear everything that people say, each one giving me different information (advice). I hear the other fencers in the auditorium yelling about their touches. I hear the machines beeping. When I lose the bout I feel relief.

AUTOGENIC PHRASES DEVELOPED FOR THIS ATHLETE

From this concentrative analysis, I developed the following autogenic phrases. From the fencer's own analysis and from observing his fencing, I knew that he was not demonstrating any specific performance problems, such as generalized anxiety at large competitions, or freezing at any particular time during the bout. Therefore, the specific phrases were constructed to enhance and reinforce his plan to fence his best.

As you will see, the phrases are taken almost directly from the fencer's almost unconscious self-talk when he fenced his best. The phrases in Part A were developed for him to use before starting his bout. They reinforce his belief in his abilities and will increase his self-confidence by affirming how well he has prepared for the competition.

AFFIRMATION OF PREPARATION

- I practiced hard.
- I trained well.
- I have taken more lessons than anytime before.
- I have beaten strong fencers before.
- I have beaten people from the best fencing countries!

The phrases in Part B will also be used before each bout. They are designed to reinforce motivation, determination, and self-belief.

Self-Confidence

- I can beat anybody!
- I know I can do it!
- I will do what I have to do get all obstacles out of my way.

On the on-guard line, Part C is used as a final mental tune-up, just before the bout begins.

Final Instructions

- I am charged, eager, and ready to go!

The self-suggestion phrases in Part D are used during the bout to focus attention, enhance concentration, and encourage relaxed alertness. They help the fencer to focus on the actions and preparations that he intends to use on the strip, encouraging active fencing (taking initiative and control). Since language is taken directly from the fencer's memory of his best performance, these phrases should also help to trigger the positive, pleasant feelings associated with his best fencing experience, and help him to fence his best more often.

During the Bout

- Get down like a tiger.
- Stay low. Concentrate! Stay loose.
- I picture my actions.
- I picture what I am going to do!
- I am in command! I am the commander. The strip, the opponent, and me!

These consciously developed autogenic self-suggestion phrases are like a mental plan. They serve as prevention against negative thoughts. The mind cannot simultaneously focus on both positive, helpful thoughts and negative, self-defeating thoughts. As negative thoughts occur from time to time, they are pushed out by the autogenic phrases.

Because this fencer needed also to improve his basic footwork, the following individual autogenic phrases were suggested as well: "*With regular practice of footwork, my fencing is improving.*" "*I can withstand long, hard footwork practices.*" "*I like to practice footwork.*"

CONCENTRATIVE ANALYSIS OF OLYMPIC MODERN PENTATHLON ATHLETE

RUNNING WHEN HE DID HIS BEST

This is a concentrative analysis of modem pentathlete Michael Gostigian performing his best in the running event. Note the emphasis that he places on controlling fatigue and aggression through focusing on breathing and rhythm.

I see the path. I look for the opponent ahead of me. I concentrate on trying to catch him. If I do so I know that I'm running fast. I do not look at my watch anymore when I'm running. I go according to how I feel. I concentrate totally on my breathing.

I go out aggressively, but hold back a little bit, too. I'm aware of my breathing and my level of oxygenation. After the first kilometer I begin to pick up speed and become slightly more aggressive getting into a steady rhythm and pace. At the 2-kilometer mark I hear the coach yelling out the times to the other athletes and I notice that I'm doing well. At the second and third kilometers I push to the threshold and in the last kilometer I go as fast as I can. The time it takes to run the final kilometer is the same as in the previous round but I am more tired.

My race plan is to start out quickly but to run with less than maximum effort. After the second kilometer I push to the threshold, and in the final kilometer I go beyond what I think I can do. I break the race into kilometers. I have good intensity in the first kilometer because I am fresh and I'm not tired. The key is to remain in control. If I go over my limit out of my comfort zone, then I will have trouble the whole race.

I always want to feel that I am in control and that I am getting stronger and stronger and not fatiguing and getting weaker and weaker. When I feel good I say to myself, *"Make sure you get out with a strong, snappy pace and stay aware of your breathing."* After 400 meters I pull back just a little bit just to work on my breathing. Then, when I get my breathing in a rhythm I truly start the race.

In the second kilometer I must be very aggressive and very confident. I begin to get more tired but I have to concentrate on my pace, being sure not to slow down. I really have to focus on pushing that threshold and it is difficult especially in the third kilometer. In every race my third kilometer is the slowest one. We run a 2-kilometer loop two times through. The speed of the first kilometer and of the third kilometer are always the same as in all my other races. The speed of the second and of the fourth kilometer are also the same as in previous races.

I generally go out in 3 minutes and 10 seconds in the first kilometer. In the second kilometer my speed is 3 minutes and 15 seconds. My third kilometer is about 3 minutes and 22 seconds. It is 10 to 12 seconds slower than my first kilometer, but I'm more tired. My fourth kilometer is about 3 minutes and 15 seconds, the same as the second kilometer. The biggest time difference is between my first and third kilometers, because I think I back off a little bit in my third kilometer so I can be a little more aggressive in my final kilometer. It is also due to being more tired In the last kilometer I am really pushing. My heart rate is 190. I am very aggressive. I give everything I have and it hurts.

I have a lot of self-talk while I run. I say things such as *"I feel good now. Let's go up one more level, get faster."* After 2 to 3 kilometers I get tired and have to be very aggressive, very positive and it starts to hurt so that the last kilometer is very uncomfortable. I say to myself, *"Come on! If you want to win you're going to have to be strong and you're going to have to give 100 percent!"* So I become very filled with winning.

My self-talk is not structured. It's just natural and it depends on how I feel. The only structured thing that I do while I am running is breathe. I try to have my breathing flow, be fluid, and control my pace.

I am calm and composed I am confident. I am aggressive, always aware of my breathing. I am thinking about 12 minutes of aggressive effort. I believe I can give a 100 percent effort through the whole race. I feel my muscles are warmed up and are ready. I feel the heat, humidity, temperature, the sunshine, my breathing. I feel the strength versus feeling fatigued, and I feel my pace increasing. To summarize, up to the first kilometer I am aggressive but controlled. In the second kilometer I pick up the pace. In the third kilometer I start to run aggressively. In the fourth kilometer I say to myself, *"Only 3 minutes to go until I finish! Come on. Go, go, go! You can do it!"*

RUNNING WHEN HE DID HE WORST

Michael's recollection of his worst running performance again emphasizes control.

When I do my worst I tend to go out too fast. The difference between performing my best and worst is being in control. Being diligent enough when I go out in the first kilometer. Not going too fast in the first kilometer because if I am too fast, even by 3 seconds, it will kill me for the rest of the race. If I go out when I am not too fit I will go too fast because I'm not aware of my level of conditioning. If I go out of my comfort zone 1 am not aware of my correct pace; if I do not keep it, if I'm too aggressive, I die. 1 must know where my comfort zone is. If I start out at 60 percent effort I will end the race at 100 percent effort. However, if I start out at 90 percent effort I will end up at 40 percent.

THE CHOSEN AUTOGENIC PHRASES

The following autogenic phrases reinforce Michael's race plan and help to maintain his focus on the task at hand-on his race plan. They are based on his race plan and on his self-talk when performing his best

- *I am aggressive and aware of my breathing. I am oxygenated.*

1 kilometer:

- *I am fresh. I am in my comfort zone. I am in control. I am getting stronger and stronger. Get out at a good and snappy pace. Be aware of your breathing. Be aggressive but controlled.*

400 meters:

- *Pull back a little bit. Work on your breathing. Get your breathing in rhythm.*

2 kilometers:

- *Be very aggressive, very confident. Concentrate on your pace. Pick up the pace. Push to the threshold.*

3 kilometers:

- *Be very aggressive. Push. Come on. You have to be very strong. You have to give 100 percent.*

4 kilometers:

- *Come on. Go. Go. Go. You can do it. Only 3 minutes to the finish. Go. Go. Go.*

RIDING WHEN HE DID HIS BEST

Here we have a concentrative analysis of Michael Gostigian's best riding performance. He emphasizes calmness, focus, and a good relationship with the horse.

I am calm and composed I look forward to testing my ability. I am smiling. I have a good attitude. I am more preoccupied with my strategy than with whether or not I have a bad horse. If I do have a bad horse, I say to myself, *"This horse and I are new to each other. Maybe I can show that I can do better with this horse than the previous rider, who rode very badly."* So I take it as a new experience and I apply my strategy to the ride. This focus is not distracted by anything. Instead of having a negative thought—that I have the worst horse—which does not help, I am just focused on my performance, looking forward to the experience.

I talk to the horse, look at him, touch him, and make him relax. I can see if the horse is nervous, if he does not bend very well on turns. I can see if I have to hold it more, or use the reins to soften his mouth so that he can move better. My attitude is very positive, very objective. There is nothing subjective about it. I am not overreacting to anything, just going and doing what I have do. I have no emotion; I am just reacting normally.

When I have a bad horse, it actually makes me aware. My arousal is heightened I make sure that I am very active in what I am doing. When 1 have a good horse, I am more passive and sometimes I do not pay enough attention. I have actually had more bad rides with a good horse. When I am not in good form, when I start to think too much, I start to get over anxious, and if I know from the previous jump that the horse is stopping before one jump all the time, I might overreact and push the horse too hard.

I try not to overreact, not to overdo it, not to override or over perform. I try to keep very calm and composed, keeping my strategy, keeping my horse together, and listening to me.

I see all the jumps around me, I go to my position, and I look. I am very calm. I see the horse and I check my equipment and make sure it is all right. I take the horse. I look for my line, for the first obstacle, and then I go.

I might see and be aware of the spectators around me, but I do not pay attention to them. I always look beyond the jump to the spot where I want to land, not at the jump itself I never look at the jump. I look beyond the jump to the landing spot.

I do not attack at the jump. I am waiting patiently. I exhale as I approach, and I look beyond the jump to the landing spot. After the jump I look at the next obstacle, the next position.

I am looking where I am going to land when I go up to the jump. When my horse goes up I always look either at the spot where I am going to land or at the next jump because then, when the horse feels me looking at where I'm going, he can change the position of his feet and, when he lands, can be in the right position.

Sometimes my problem is that my focus is very narrow. I look at the jump and I see just the jump and for some reason I become very tense. The tension is in my hands and in my stomach.

I am very soft, loose at the shoulders. I feel my lower leg on the horse and my unlocked knees and hips. I feel the horse bending to my leg. I feel the horse in my soft fingers. My eyes are soft. I have a soft focus.

I can hear the horse breathing, the sound of his feet galloping. I can hear the noise of the obstacles when they are hit or touched by a horse. Otherwise, I do not hear anything. I do not hear people.

I always breathe like the horse because the horse relaxes when he hears it. And if it doesn't relax the horse, it relaxes me, and that in turn relaxes the horse.

I feel my legs on the horse. My lower leg is around the horse. My knees are not tensing the horse. I am very soft and I have a good rhythm, a soft rhythm and the horse is responding to me and just flowing under me.

My legs are very flexible and they are pulsing-moving back and forth with the horse-instead of squeezing, which tightens up the horse. My shoulders stay back. I have a natural leverage. I feel no tension. Just a little in the upper body to keep the horse back. I am breathing in a very good rhythm. I trust the horse. I am flowing and clear-minded.

I keep my breathing flowing with no expectation that the horse will stop before the jump, because that makes me stop breathing. I just keep the breathing going and I think the horse feels it. I always feel tension in my stomach, and my heart rate is pretty high (140-150).

My strategy is to always be in control, telling the horse, "*Whoa,*" and "*wait for the jump.*" Based on what I learn about the horse, my strategy is generally not to hurry, not to be impatient, not to attack, just wait for the jump and be calm. I just pretend that the obstacles are not there, because everything in riding is between the obstacles, what I do between the obstacles, and in the control. And if I can get the horse back and under control, all I have to do is have a good balance and the jumps take care of themselves automatically.

All I have to do is just plan ahead and look for the next obstacle. That is my basic strategy and it works for all horses. Some horses need more leg work, other horses need more control, to be held back. I talk to the horse. *"Whoa." "Relax, whoa." "Calm, slow."*

I say to myself, *"Wait, wait. I am waiting, I am waiting. I just have to wait, and trust the horse. I do not have to hurry."* If I push the horse with my legs, then I am hurrying. Many times I see the landing spot and I rush to go, to hurry up, because of my anxiety. If I have fear, I think the horse will stop before the jump and I push. This is my problem-anxiety.

I just have to trust the horse and think the obstacles are not there that it is just on the way.

Sometimes I say to myself, *"Wait, wait,"* and in the last moment I change my self-talk and get anxious, impatient, and I go, and this is the problem.

So if I say to myself, *"I am coming into the turn, the corner. OK, hold it, re-group, keep the balance, breathe again, recover, and go to the next jump."*

Some horses like to go close for the jump and I have to wait. Some like a farther take-off spot. That is why I do not look at the take-off spot.

If I make a mistake, I say, *"Forget about it, look for the next obstacle. Forget it and try to get the horse back in balance."*

My arousal level is high, 10 on a scale of 1 to 10.

RIDING WHEN PERFORMING HIS WORST

When I ride my worst, everything is the same. Only one thing is different: I break my concentration on my plan. All it takes is one mistake. I hurry and I attack the jump. The horse gets fast I lose the balance, and I start making mistakes. Then I usually re-group, but the horse changes and makes mistakes. I have to re-group immediately and slow down and wait, taking total control.

When I ride my worst, everything is too fast. I have no control. I have fear of knocking down the obstacles. 1 do not trust the horse and then I overreact. I am impatient, not composed, anxious.

I have fear of stopping the horse. I have narrow focus. I am looking only at the jump. I am not breathing. I am pinching the horse with my knees. 1 go too fast. I am too strong with my hands. I am hitting the jump. I am not waiting or sitting up. I abandon my riding tactics.

THE CHOSEN AUTOGENIC PHRASES

Again these phrases are designed as a reinforcement of his race plan-keeping the focus on the task at hand.

- *I am looking forward to this challenge, to this new experience.*
- *I had excellent training performances this year—I am confident.*
- *I recall my training and positive feelings from Radnor Hunt Club.*
- *I feel good.*
- *Calm and confident.*
- *See, touch, talk to the horse.*
- *Be gentle to the horse.*
- *I am a new rider. I can show that this horse can do better than he did for the previous rider, who rode very badly.*
- *I am soft, loose, relaxed. I am one with the horse.*
- *Calm and composed.*
- *Breathe like a horse.*
- *Talk to the horse.*
- *Focus on the landing spot.*
- *Wait patiently.*
- *Exhale before the obstacle.*

- *Plan ahead. Look at the next obstacle.*
- *Breathing soft, eyes soft, soft fingers.*
- *Clear mind. Focus on each jump.*
- *I am coming into the turn. Okay, hold it. Re-group. Keep the balance. Breathing again. Recover and go to the next jump. Talk to the horse: "Whoa," "Relax, whoa, Calm, slow." Trust the horse, wait.*
- *Forget about it! Look for the next obstacle.*

SWIMMING WHEN HE DID HIS BEST

The following is the concentrative analysis of Michael Gostigian's best swimming performance. Notice how much he concentrates on his breathing.

I get on the block. Then I look down and I just see my lane-50 meters. I say to myself "*50 meters six times is 300 meters. So I am going to be very aggressive, and make sure I make six good laps.*"

I see the blue water and the flags. I hear the judge.

When I swim I do not see anything, just the line and the wall. I do not see anybody or anything. It takes about 20 strokes to do 50 meters. After 20 strokes I look up and see the wall I make my turn. Around the 16 to 20 stoke point I am looking for the wall, getting to the wall, making a good turn, coming up, and then getting faster-

I do not hear anything. Maybe the water splashing on my ears. I feel the pressure of the water and I feel my strokes. But I do not hear any people. I do not even see my opponents.

I feel control. I feel strength. I feel my strength with each stroke. I feel my breathing. At critical moments when I am swimming I try to feel my stomach moving up and down when I breathe. When I feel my mark-which is halfway through the race-I really start to work mentally. I actually start my race here, really concentrating on what I am doing.

I do not really think during the race. It is all just self-talk: "*Come on,*" "*That's the 125 meter mark,*" "*Start to do this.*" "*Getting more aggressive, getting the strokes longer.*"

At the 200 meter mark I say to myself, "*100 meters to go! Start kicking hard,*" so I start kicking harder.

Then it's "*Fifty meters to go,*" and "*Full stretch, very aggressive!*" and I just concentrate on very long strokes, and on very strong kicking.

When there are just 25 meters left and I feel dead, I just think about how much I want to win. At the last 12 meter mark I am very much aware that I do not want to breathe, just swim, because if l turn my head and breathe I lose time and my form. I usually feel pain at the last 40 meters. It hurts, really hurts. The last 25 meters every stroke hurts. I have high determination. I am aggressive, not afraid I am confident in myself due to good preparation. I know I am the best in the world. It is my sport.

SWIMMING WHEN HE DID HIS WORST

My confidence is low. If I swim my worst my confidence is low because my preparation, my training was not good This is the only reason my confidence is low, because I know that I did not do the work.

Sometimes I hold my breath because of the anxiety and go out too fast. I do not have patience because of my anxiety. I do not keep my race plan. If there is any time that I make mistakes (I do it very rarely) it is that I go out too fast in the first 100 meters.

Sometimes I went out too easy, too relaxed, not aggressive enough, too passive. (there may be something at the bottom of the page that I cannot read). I feel tired, scared, weak, and hurt.

THE CHOSE AUGTOGENIC PHRASES

Once more, autogenic phrases are like a race plan helping to maintain the focus on the task at hand.

- *I am in control.*
- *My muscles are flexible and loose.*
- *My strokes are smooth. I feel strength with each stroke.*
- *I feel my breathing! I feel my stomach moving up and down. My stomach is loose, my breathing is fluid and natural.*

100 meters:

- *Long, smooth strokes, but aggressive!*

125 meters:

- *That is the 125 meter mark, get more aggressive, longer strokes!*

200 meters:

- *100 meters to go!*
- *Get on your race plan!*
- *Change the tempo!*
- *Change from first to second gear!*

300 meters:

- *Very aggressive, very aggressive!*
- *Maintain the rhythm!*

Last 50 meters:

- *Reach even more!*
- *50 meters to go-use your legs.*
- *Full stretch, very aggressive!*
- *Long strokes, very strong kicking!*

Last 12 meters:

- *Stop breathing!*
- *Go!*
- *I am the best.*
- *It is my sport.*

Suggestions for Preparing for the Competition

- Develop a mindset filled with love of playing the game (sport) and love of the challenge. Focus your mind set on the pleasure of going for it, on the challenge, instead of having a mindset of avoiding errors and failure, which only assures errors and failure.

- Appreciate the joy playing totally free from fear.

- Remember your life and performances are greatly influenced by your habits of thinking. You must have good thoughts and you must implement them.

- Stop worrying, ruminating about past and future events. Do not dwell on mistakes or on a bad play, action, because it will affect your entire game. Focus on your game and immerse yourself totally in what you are doing.

- Get ready for the competition mentally as well as physically.

- Have a mental race (performance) plan. This will help you to concentrate on the task at hand.

- One game, play, shot, touch at a time! Be on the present, avoid dwelling on past and future events. Do not dwell on your errors or mistakes.

- Stay calm inside. Do not get angry with yourself, have positive thoughts.

- Be relaxed; physical tension begins in the mind. Control your thoughts.

- Believe in yourself and you will be more calm.

- Be always positive, never say I cannot do it.

- If you can win in your mind, you can win in the competition. Never think about losing.

- Be self-confident. If you are afraid and insecure, the opponent will feel it. You influence your opponent. Evaluate your chances realistically but add 15 percent to the positive side. Believe in yourself, but do not be overconfident.

- Be in a good mood. Positive emotions make your performance better, develops physiological changes in your body.
- Be happy. Your mind, mood influence your body. Think about pleasant things, pleasant outcomes.

REMINDERS IN CONSTRUCTING YOUR TRAINING AND COMPETITION ROUTINE

Now you know the common asanas that can be assimilated into athletic training and how to put them together. Here are some things to keep in mind as you begin to practice.

- Breath is the link between your body and mind. The state of your breathing reflects the state of your mind. It is the primary vehicle for bringing energy (prana) into your body. Use breathing to balance the interaction between body and mind and to stabilize your emotional energy. Through awareness and control of your breath and the energy (prana) within it, you can get conscious control over your body's physiological systems.
- When you are facing a difficult situation, take a long, slow, deep breath, and exhale slowly, releasing the tension from your body.
- When you make an error or mistake, or are confused, take a moment to re-focus and re-group. Ground yourself in breath awareness. Focus on the smoothness and evenness of your breath, eliminating all jerks and pauses. A few moments of calm breathing will help you overcome intense emotion. Practice daily to learn to calm your breathing.
- In the competition, as pressure increases, use your breath to stay focused on the task at hand. Chest breathing automatically increases activity within your nervous system. If you notice tension, chase it away by breathing evenly and

diaphragmatically. Always monitor your breathing patterns to be sure you are breathing from your diaphragm.

- If your arousal level is too high, use breathing with prolonged exhalation. Slow down the rate of exhalation until you are exhaling for twice as long as you are inhaling. By contracting your abdomen, you will help prolong the exhalation. Do not try to fill or empty your lungs completely—just simply change the rhythm of your breath. Visualize the air entering through the nostrils and then leaving through the nostrils as you exhale. Focus on the smoothness and evenness of your breath. A few moments of calm breathing will help you overcome high arousal, intense emotion.

- If your arousal level is too low, if you feel "flat," to mobilize yourself take a few short breaths. It will immediately enliven your body and spirit.

- Use alternate nostril breathing to calm, balance, and to regulate energy on physical as well as subtle levels. Alternate nostril breathing eliminate wastes, and strengthens the nerves leading to stability, tranquillity and clarity of mind. Each nostril has a different effect on the mind and body. The right nostril activates and warms. It intensifies the activity of the body and mind. It is preferred to breathe through this nostril while eating, conducting business or participating in sports. The left nostril has a receptive, cooling influence and is preferable to use while listening, studying, resting, and renewing the body and mind.

- Use the Double "R" breath to regroup, re-focus.

- Be aware that in spite of the many positive physiological effects of asanas, they are only a means to achieve the main goal—to facilitate meditation and calm the disturbances of the mind. Yoga Sutras contains 200 aphorisms. Only 3 deal with asanas, the rest deals with meditation.

- If you are tired, do some yoga asanas (YRE). These will help you speed up the recovery process, loosening up the tight muscles.

- Starting your daily training, competition with a yoga routine described in the previous chapters will clear your mind and help you remain focused.
- Remember that yoga exercises must be supported by a healthy diet. Without, it will not be useful. Food can destroy or sustain your body.
- Practice TM. Meditation purifies the mind, strengthens your nervous system, and clears your mind. A clear mind knows what to say, what word to use, using the right tone and body language.
- Calmness is the best way to deal with problems.
- Remember, there is a quiet, safe place you can go to without paying a penny. That place is within you! You can take advantage of this place to return for recharging your energy, calming your turbulent thoughts, and experiencing silence.

  Sit in a comfortable position. Relax your whole body.

  Be aware of your breathing. Do not change it. Let it flow naturally in your own rhythm. Focus on the space where the air enters and leaves your nostrils. Listen to your breathing.

  Focus your attention on your solar plexus.

  Attune to the solar plexus and to your breathing.

  Remain in this position for several minutes attuning, to your solar plexus and to the silence.

  Use this exercise every day to calm and recharge yourself. You can use it also in a competition during breaks.
- Remember, suggestion and faith is the essence of healing! Have faith! It is a potent force. Believe in yourself, in your goals and ideas.
- Concentrate! Whatever you do, put everything into it.
- Remember, your performances and your life are very much influenced by your thoughts. You must have positive thoughts and you must implement them.
- The ability to stay focused on positive thoughts is what separates successful athletes from non-successful ones.

- The key to getting control of your mind in a competition is being able to re-focus, to get the negative thoughts out. For example, if a negative thought came through, you simply re-focus to some positive thought you use when performing your best.

- It is important to rebound yourself from a bad game, action, shoot, etc. Do not dwell on errors and mistakes. Drop the negative thought and re-focus. Combine re-focusing with relaxation and positive self-talk.

- To re-focus, drop the negative thought. Relax, use the Double "R" breathing and immediately re-focus on the task at hand, and on positive thoughts. Use the prepared autogenic phrases (see Chapter 15) simultaneously. This will help you stop worrying and ruminating about past and future events.

- Focus on your game plan and immerse yourself totally in what you are doing. Play one game at a time. Be in the present, do not dwell on mistakes. The play that matters is the one you are playing. Thinking about the future play and results is self-defeating.

- Be relaxed. Physical tension begins in the mind. Control your thoughts. When you are calm mentally, you will be also physically relaxed. Believe in yourself and you will be more calm.

- Shut out everything around you when competing. One of my fencers recalled his self-talk from his best performance: *"I see only the strip, the opponent, and me."* A golfer may say, *"The green, the ball, and my club."*

- Remember that getting ready for the competition is mental as well as physical.

- Have a free, natural, confident attitude. Feel good. Focus on the pleasure of going for it, or the challenge, instead of mind set of avoiding errors and failure which leads to errors and failure.

- Believe and trust yourself. Go for your goals. Enjoy the challenge.

- Always be positive. Never say, "I cannot do it." Remind yourself that pressure is self-imposed, self-induced. Pressure is something you put on yourself. The stimuli, conditions, and what is happening are not important. How we react and respond to what happens is important.

- Stress occurs when you believe you are unable to solve a problem.

- Awareness is the first step to manage stress. Make a list of things that worry you, that are causing stress. This will be the starting point to develop coping skills to manage your stress level.

- Your coping skills strategies will include breathing exercises and relaxation techniques to control the somatic aspect of stress and self-talk, and positive affirmations to control the cognitive aspect of stress.

- Focus on what you can control and forget things that you cannot. Remember that successful persons differ from unsuccessful persons. The successful person failed and tried again, when the second merely failed.

- Enjoy the experience of what you are doing, whether it is study, sports, playing with your children, or competing for the Olympic gold medal. If you enjoy your experience, your involvement, you are free and in control of what you are doing. If the main reward is the enjoyment, experiencing the involvement, activity, the sport, you will become free, happy and you will improve your performance and ultimately your life.

- Enjoyment is in the process of improvement and happiness is in the process of self-exploration, self-knowledge—knowing your inner self, which is divine.

APPENDIX A ━━━
ERICKSON'S UTILIZATION
APPROACH TO AT

The traditional AT approach involves a psychologist suggesting to a subject that he or she feel a certain way. The psychologist indicates directly what the subject should experience. For example, "Your arms are heavy, very heavy."

In contrast, techniques evolving from the works of the late Milton Erickson, M.D., may be described as following an anthropological rather than the "missionary" approach of traditional AT (Feldman, 1985). Instead of directing the individual according to a pre-set series of formulas or instructions, the psychologist joins with the person, adapting to and utilizing the individual's ongoing experience. Each person is viewed as unique and is expected to experience the autogenic state in his or her own way.

The Erickson technique involves providing options. For example:

> "You may have a heavy feeling or a light feeling in your arms,

or

> "You may experience a warm, pleasant feeling or a tingling sensation."

The method acknowledges the content and pacing of the individual's responses, and the subject is led toward further alternatives. The essential element of this process of pacing and leading involves the acceptance and utilization of whatever autogenic phenomena the individual experiences and, thus, the Ericksonian approach is often termed the Utilization Approach.

When a psychologist practices AT, he or she can individualize it to the athlete's needs and resources. The psychologist can also provide options and alternatives by utilizing the athlete's own experience of relaxation and by guiding and encouraging individualized imagery rather than giving instruction to relax. If, for example, in the first basic AT exercise, the athlete experiences the sensation of lightness when he or she relaxes, the verbal suggestion, *"The arms are heavy"* is inadequate and confusing. Using the Utilization Approach, an alternative instruction is:

> *"I wonder if you can be conscious about the changing sensations in your arms as you relax and become comfortable."*

And then,

> *"You may feel heaviness or lightness in your arms."*

In addition to indirectly suggesting that the individual will relax and feel more comfortable, this approach allows the psychologist and the subject to co-create the experience in a way that enhances the individual's perception of the changing sensations that accompany the altered state. Also, because the suggestions are embedded within a larger sentence structure designed to arouse and challenge curiosity, the individual tends not to be consciously aware of the psychologist's suggestions to be relaxed and comfortable.

Additional alternative phrases for the introductory AT relaxation exercises include:

> *"I wonder whether you can be aware of how your breathing becomes deeper, easier, and more regular as your diaphragm muscles relax."*
>
> *"We might be curious about the sensations that develop in your arms, whether they feel heavy, as many people feel just sinking in the chair, or if they feel lighter and lighter."*
>
> *"That's right, as the muscles relax the circulation increases, which makes the arms feel warm."*

These statements demonstrate that this method offers options and alternatives. The athlete's own experiences of relaxation and individualized creative imagery are used rather than the instruction to relax. This approach deepens the relaxation and enhances the sensations which occur.

APPENDIX B ━━━
PRACTICE SCHEDULE FOR AT

Each day, write down every time that you practice AT. Record your feelings about the experience and describe any surprises. Also evaluate each practice session using the following scale.

Evaluation scale: +2 = very good; +1 = more good than bad; 0 = neither good nor bad- -1 = more bad than good; -2 = very bad

Practice Date	Practice No.	Feelings/ Experiences	Evaluation

Appendix C ■■■■■
AT for Rapid Switch-off
and Recovery

Sometimes the athlete must accomplish a rapid and complete switch-off. The following is another example of a procedure for rapid switch-off and recovery used in the Olympic Games in Seoul by one of the author's students during brief breaks in the competition.

Each muscle is relaxed.

I am totally calm.

Each muscle is relaxed.

I am totally calm.

Each muscle is relaxed.

I am totally calm.

Each muscle is relaxed.

I am totally calm.

My whole body is heavy, very heavy.

My limbs are like lead.

I am totally calm, totally switched off.

My breath is calm and regular.

And my heartbeat is very strong.

My breath is calm and regular and my heartbeat is strong.

I feel strong, fresh, and my whole body is refreshed.

Strength is returning to my limbs.

I am again preparing to compete.

Deep breath.

Open eyes.

Stretch.

Appendix D
AT for Stress Release Before Competition

This routine for Autogenic Training, prepared by A.V. Alekseyev, was used successfully in the Olympic Games in Montreal, Moscow, and Seoul by Czechoslovakian and U.S. athletes:

- I am calm. I am beginning to feel relaxed. I am free from all inner tension. I am indifferent to all worries, all concerns are far away. I feel deep relaxation. I am totally calm.

- Now I focus my attention on my face. I visualize it. My face is smooth and calm. My entire body is calm. My attention is totally focused on my face. My face is calm, smooth, and motionless. (The athlete should visualize all this, feel that it is happening, and let it happen.)

- I switch my attention to my arms and hands. I visualize them. My arms and hands feel relaxed and warm. My hands and fingers are relaxed and warm. My forearms and elbows are relaxing and becoming warm. My shoulders and neck are relaxing and becoming warm. Both arms are relaxed and warm. I feel the wave of warmth moving from my shoulders down to my fingers.

- I switch my attention to my face. My face is calm and motionless. My entire body is calm and motionless.

- I switch my attention to my legs. I visualize them. My legs are beginning to relax and are becoming warm. My feet, calves, and knees are relaxing and becoming warm. My thighs and hips are relaxing and becoming warm. Both legs are relaxed and warm. I feel the wave of warmth flowing down all the way to my toes. (The athlete should visualize all this and feel that is happening.)

- I switch my attention to my face. My face is calm and motionless. I switch my attention to the trunk of my body. I visualize it. The trunk of my body is totally relaxed and warm.

- My attention is focused on my chest. My breathing is calm and easy.

- My attention is focused on my heart. My heartbeat is strong and regular. My heart is resting.

- I switch my attention to my face. My face is calm and motionless. My entire body is calm and motionless. I am at rest. I have rested, I have become calm, and my entire body has regenerated. I have regained my strength. I have reenergized my body. I feel strong.

APPENDIX E ━━━━━━━

EXAMPLE OF AT FOR ENERGY RECOVERY, POSITIVE ATTITUDE

The following phrases, prepared by A.V. Alekseyev, have proven beneficial for recovery after hard training. They are also useful for increasing self-assurance, satisfaction, and positive attitude during periods of intense training.

- **Calmness.** I am calm. I am beginning to feel relaxed. I am free from all inner tension. I am totally calm. I feel deeply relaxed.

- **Relaxation.** Now I take three deep breaths and let go. With each deep breath I take, I will relax more and more. My breathing is calm and easy. My entire body is calm and relaxed. My breathing is calm and regular.

- **Arms.** Now I turn my attention to my arms. I visualize them. My arms are beginning to relax and are becoming warm. My forearms and elbows feel relaxed and pleasantly warm. My shoulders and my neck are relaxing and becoming warm. The muscles of both my arms are relaxed, limp, and soft. I feel a wave of warmth pouring from my shoulders down to my fingertips. (The athlete should visualize all this and feel that it is happening.)

- **Breathing**. Now I switch my attention to my breathing. My breathing is easy and regular.

- **Legs**. I turn my attention to my legs. I visualize them. My legs are beginning to relax and are becoming warm. My feet, calves, and knees are relaxed and pleasantly warm. My thighs and knees are relaxed and pleasantly warm. My thighs and hips are relaxed and warm. The muscles of both my legs are relaxed, limp, and soft. I feel a wave of warmth pouring all the way to my toes.

- **Breathing and Calmness.** I switch my attention to my breathing. My breathing is regular and calm. My whole body is calm. I am at rest.

- **Hips/Chest/Abdomen.** I turn my attention to my hips, chest, and abdomen. I visualize them. My hips, chest, and abdomen are totally relaxed and warm. The muscles of my back, the muscles of my entire trunk, are relaxed and warm. (The athlete should visualize this and let it happen.) My attention is focused on my chest. My breathing is calm and easy.

- **Heart.** My attention is focused on my heart. My heartbeat is strong and regular. My heart is resting. My whole body is at rest.

- **Face.** I focus attention on my face. The muscles of my face are smooth and calm. My entire body is calm.

- **Recovery.** My whole body feels quiet, comfortable, and rested. I feel refreshed.

- **Motivation.** I trained hard. I feel good about myself I am willing to do in each workout what I have to do to reach my goal. I am prepared to extend myself in each practice.

- **Confidence.** I believe in myself. I believe in my capacity to achieve my goal. I am confident.

- **Positive Attitude.** Achieving my goal requires daily effort. I am prepared. I am in an excellent mood. I am ready to train again.

- **Activation/Readiness.** I feel good. I am at rest and am regaining my strength. The sensation of heaviness is disappearing from my arms and legs and from my entire body.

All my muscles are becoming light and elastic. My feeling of drowsiness has disappeared. I am feeling more and more fresh. I take a deep breath. My head is clear. My mood is good and fresh. I am at full strength. I am ready to act. Stand up. Exercise the arms. I feel refreshed, reenergized, and confident. I am again ready to train.

APPENDIX F ━━━━
A SAMPLE TRAINING PROGRAM

In Chapters 14 and 15, you learned AT. AT is a particularly effective technique since you simultaneously practice three mental skills: relaxation, concentration, and imagery. The relaxation during AT is achieved through concentration. AT is also helpful in stimulating imagery and in focusing attention. My students after learning AT create their own individual specific AT, and/or use the basic AT for relaxation.

The advantage of AT is that it involves not only the musculoskeletal system, but also the autonomic and cognitive processes. AT fosters a type of self-reliance as well. From the start the athlete has a clear and simple procedure that he or she can use on his or her own. AT by its nature involves self-control. It is distinguished by the fact that it places the responsibility for the athlete's growth and performance not on a coach or psychologist or technician, but on the athlete himself or herself.

So, by practicing daily AT, the athlete also practices and improves concentration.

In the 1993 NCAA championships, my students' warm-up looked very different from those of the other fencers. They also behaved differently during the breaks between bouts by practicing AT and yoga regeneration exercises. Ben Atkins, 1993 NCAA epee champion (also 1991 NCAA foil champion) and his NCAA team champion teammate Mark Pavese, start each training session or competition with "sitting still" and "concentrating on breathing" for 2 to 3 minutes. This brief exercise is a mental tune up for them.

They then use two simple yoga postures as concentration exercises during warm-ups: Forward Bend; and Seated Forward Bend. The focal point during both yoga postures is on the hamstrings and on the muscles of the back—the physiological effect of the postures. These exercises are also both a mental and physical tune-up for them.

Although these yoga exercises take only a few minutes, Mark and Ben find them very useful in shifting themselves from a usual state of awareness to a more focused, concentrated state. They serve as a transition to the concentration, which is so important during competition and training. They are now mentally ready to concentrate on their fencing. After finishing their concentration exercises, they continue with their regular warm-up routine.

Immediately after training or competition, my students do 3 to 4 Yoga Regenerative Exercises, which speed up the process of regeneration and serve also for prevention of injury. The focal point during these exercises is on deactivation and relaxation—the psychological effect of the yoga exercises. They terminate the training with AT.

Michael Gostigian, U.S. National Pentathlon Champion and member of the 1988 and 1992 U.S. Olympic Pentathlon team, uses the same Yoga postures to practice concentration and to warm-up as Ben and Mark. However, Michael uses different yoga recovery exercises, because his athletic demands of his sport are different from those of Ben and Mark.

As with AT, yoga exercises are extremely efficient. In a short period of time, you can simultaneously accomplish several training tasks. Selecting a yoga exercise during warm-up serves two functions at once. It is a means for practicing attention and concentration and it is also a warm-up for the body. You can simultaneously improve flexibility, body awareness, self-control, and relaxation. Yoga exercises can also speed up the process of recovery.

In addition, yoga concentration exercises are a transition into the concentration that you need during training and competition. One becomes accustomed to concentrating while warming up physically. It is easier to stay motivated for yoga exercises than for other concentration exercises.

Yoga helps develop the habit of fully concentrating on what you are doing. Literally, yoga concentration becomes as much a part of the routine as the daily stretching. Practicing concentration becomes a habit when done regularly and systematically and when combined with the basic physical routine.

After learning the four basic steps, my students practice daily mediation or at least breath awareness.

GLOSSARY ▬▬▬

ABDOMINAL BREATHING. diaphragm breathing

ALTERNATE NOSTRIL BREATHING. alternating inhalation and exhalation through different nostrils

ASANA. body posture

AUTOGENIC PHRASES. "self talk"; repeated phrases in the mind

AUTOGENIC TRAINING (AT). autoregulatory system involves relaxation and concentration; mind-body training system

BASIC AUTOGENIC (EXERCISES) PHRASES. heaviness, warmth, calm breathing, cardiac (heartbeat) solar plexus, cool forehead

CONCENTRATION. attention focus on the task at hand

CONCENTRATIVE ANALYSIS. in a trance state recalling vividly one's best performance and later one's worst performance

COORDINATION TENSION. occurs when an individual is learning new movements or skills; unwanted tension occurs

DHARANA. concentration on one object, idea

DHYANA. meditation, steady concentration on one object, idea

HATHA YOGA. Exercises for the body consisting of asanas, pranayama, relaxation and cleansing techniques

IDEOMOTOR TRAINING. East European term for utilization imagery in sports; literally means imagining of a certain movement, skill, or action in order to improve it

IDEOMOTOR SET-UP. a psychological factor that relates to movement; it is one of the main elements in determining the form, structure of a movement

INDIVIDUAL-SPECIFIC AUTOGENIC PHRASES. similar to posthypnotic suggestions in hypnosis

INDIVIDUALLY TAILORED AT. AT designed individually based on specific needs

KINESTHETIC TRAINING. training oneself in body awareness and muscular tension; means isometric contraction of a certain muscle group with varying degrees (effort) and then total relaxation of muscles

PASSIVE CONCENTRATION. attention focus without strain or effort, with a non-striving attitude; "let it happen"; gateway for controlling autonomic involuntary functions

PRANAYAMA. breathing exercises

PRATYAHARA. control of senses; sense withdrawal; a final preparation for meditation

RELAXATION. "not doing"; allowing the muscles to decrease tension

SAMADHI. a state of super-consciousness; the individual self is united with the universal self

SCHULTZ'S CLASSICAL AT. consists of six categories of exercise. muscle, blood vessels, heart, breathing, organs of the stomach, and forehead

SELF-STUDY, SELF-EDUCATION. lifelong process to develop one's physical mental, intellectual, and moral qualities

SPEED TENSION. occurs especially in movements that are executed at maximum speed; under these conditions, muscles are not able to relax completely

SPORT-MODIFIED AT. AT applied to sport, athletes

TONIC TENSION. increased level of tension in muscles in the resting state due to stress and anxiety

TRAINING DIARY. tool in self-study

YAMA AND NIYAMA. moral, ethical, and health guidelines

YOGA COMPENSATION EXERCISES (YCE). exercises to correct and compensate for the developed muscle dysbalance due to "one-sided" training and/or overloading certain muscle groups

YOGA REGENERATION EXERCISES (YRE). biological process fostered by athlete for regaining strength and prevention of injury; means for speeding up the recovery process

YOGA SUPPLEMENTAL EXERCISES (YSE). sports and activities other than one's sport in order to build overall fitness

YOGA SUTRAS. the first written synthesis of yoga from the second century B.C.

BIBLIOGRAPHY

Baktay, E. *A Diadalmas Jóga*. Budapest: Pantheon, 1942.

Ben-Menachem, M. *A Ben-Menachem Szugesztio*. Budapest Courier, Reszvenytarsasag, 1992.

Boytov, V.G. and A.D. Movsovitch. *The Willpower of Young Fencers as a Prerequisite of Their Successful Fencing*. Toria and Practica Fyzkult, 1976.

Bytechnina, Tysler, Pashkevitch. *The Psychological Aspect of Offensive Actions of Fencers*. Teoria and Practica Fyzkult, 1976.

Carr, Rachel. *The Yoga Way to Release Tension*. New York: Barnes and Noble Books, 1974.

Chopra, Deepak, M.D. *Ageless Body Timeless Mind*. New York: Harmony Books, 1993.

------------. *Quantum Healing*. New York: Bantam Books, 1989.

Christensen, Alice. *The American Yoga Association Beginner's Manual*. New York: Simon and Schuster, 1987.

Dely, K. *Joga Gyakorlatak*. Budapest: Sport, 1973.

Fair, P. *Biofeedback Principles and Practice for Clinicians*. Edited by J. Basmajian, M.D. Williams and Williams, 1983.

Gach, Michael Reed, with Carolyn Marco. *Acu-Yoga*. Japan Publications, 1981.

Jesuidan, Selva Raja. *Sport és Joga.* Budapest: Pantheon, 1942.

Kabat-Zinn, Jon. *Full Catastrophe Living.* New York: Dell Publishing Group, 1990.

Kogler, A. *Clearing the Path to Victory: A Self-Guided Mental Training Program for Athletes.* Lansdowne, Pennsylvania: Counterparry Press, 1994.

------------. "Ideomotor Training." 1968.

------------. *Joga*, Telesne Cvicenia, Dychanie, Autogenny Training. Bratislva: Sport, Slovenske Telovychovne Vydavatelstvo, 1971.

------------. *Joga.* Bratislva: Sport, Slovenske Telovychovne Vydavatelstvo, 1978.

------------. "The Effect of Ideomotor Training in learning and Remembering Gymnastic Kill." Acta Facultatis Educationis Physicae Universistatis Comenianae, SPN Bratislava. 1971.

------------. "The Influence of a Combined Method of Ideomotor and Practical Training on the Speed of a Direct Thrust with Lunge and Advance-Lunge, and on the Acquisition of Fundmentals in Fencing." Theor. Praxe Tel. Vych. 24, 1976, 9.

------------. "The Influence of Combined Method of Ideomotor and Practical Training in Learning Applied to Diving." Teor Praxe Tel. Vych. 23, 1975.

------------. "The Effect of Combined Method of Ideomotor and Practical Training in Learning Gymnastic Motor Skill with 16-18-year-old Boys." Teor Praxe Tel. Vych. 16, 1968.

------------. *Preparing the Mind.* Lansdowne, Pennsylvania: Counterparry Press, 1993.

Orme-Johnsons, D.W. and J.T. Farrow. *Scientific Research on the Transcendental Meditation Program, Collected Papers.* Vol. 1. Meru Press, 1976.

Peper, E.,M. Guinn, and S. Ancoli. *Mind-Body Integration.* New York: Plenum Press, 1979.

Pribram, K. *Neuropsychology of Achievement*. Sybervision System, 1985.

Puni, A.C. "Psychologie Sportu." Lectures of the Institute of Physical Education and Sport. Prague, 1957.

Roth, Robert. *Maharishi Mahesh Yogi's TM*. New York: Donald I. Fine, 1987.

Schultz, J.H. *Das Autogene Training*. Stuttgart, Thieme, 1966.

Swami Rama. *Inspired Thoughts of Swami Rama*. Homesdale, Pennsylvania: The Himalayan International Institute of Yoga Science and Philosophy of the U.S.A., 1983.

------------. *Lectures on Yoga*. Homesdale, Pennsylvania: The Himalayan International Institute of Yoga Science and Philosophy of the U.S.A,. 1988.

------------. *Living with the Himalayan Masters*. Homesdale Pennsylvania: The Himalayan International Institute of Yoga Science and Philosophy of the U.S.A., 1978.

------------. *Meditation and Its Practice*. Homesdale, Pennsylvania: The Himalayan International Institute of Yoga Science and Philosophy of the U.S.A., 1992.

Swami Rama. *Science of Breath*. Homesdale, Pennsylvania:The Himalayan International Institute of Yoga Science and Philosophy of the U.S.A., 1979.

Swami Sivananda Radha. *Hatha Yoga, The Hidden Language*. Boston: Shambhala Publications, Inc., 1987.

Thomas, K. *Praxis der Selbsthypnose des Autogenen Trainings*. Stuttgart: Georg Thieme. 1976.

Vigh, B. A *Joga És Az Idegrendszer*. Budapest: Gondolat Kiadó, 1980.

------------. *Joga Es Tudomany*. Budapest: Gondolat, 1972.

Weninger, A. *A Keleti Joga*. Budapest: Vörösvari, 1943.

INDEX

On the following pages you will find listed, with their current prices, some of the books now available on related subjects. Your book dealer stocks most of these and will stock new titles in the Llewellyn series as they become available. We urge your patronage.

TO GET A FREE CATALOG

You are invited to write for our bi-monthly news magazine/catalog, *Llewellyn's New Worlds of Mind and Spirit*. A sample copy is free, and it will continue coming to you at no cost as long as you are an active mail customer. Or you may subscribe for just $10 in the United States and Canada ($20 overseas, first class mail). Many bookstores also have *New Worlds* available to their customers. Ask for it.

In *New Worlds* you will find news and features about new books, tapes and services; announcements of meetings and seminars; helpful articles; author interviews and much more. Write to:

Llewellyn's New Worlds of Mind and Spirit
P.O. Box 64383-K387, St. Paul, MN 55164-0383, U.S.A.

TO ORDER BOOKS AND TAPES

If your book store does not carry the titles described on the following pages, you may order them directly from Llewellyn by sending the full price in U.S. funds, plus postage and handling (see below).

Credit card orders: VISA, MasterCard, American Express are accepted. Call us toll-free within the United States and Canada at 1-800-THE-MOON.

Special Group Discount: Because there is a great deal of interest in group discussion and study of the subject matter of this book, we offer a 20% quantity discount to group leaders or agents. Our Special Quantity Price for a minimum order of five copies of *Yoga for Every Athlete* is $67.80 cash-with-order. Include postage and handling charges noted below.

Postage and Handling: Include $4 postage and handling for orders $15 and under; $5 for orders *over* $15. There are no postage and handling charges for orders over $100. Postage and handling rates are subject to change. We ship UPS whenever possible within the continental United States; delivery is guaranteed. Please provide your street address as UPS does not deliver to P.O. boxes. Orders shipped to Alaska, Hawaii, Canada, Mexico and Puerto Rico will be sent via first class mail. Allow 4-6 weeks for delivery. **International orders:** Airmail – add retail price of each book and $5 for each non-book item (audiotapes, etc.); Surface mail – add $1 per item.

Minnesota residents add 7% sales tax.

Mail orders to:
Llewellyn Worldwide, P.O. Box 64383-K387, St. Paul, MN 55164-0383, U.S.A.

For customer service, call (612) 291-1970.

THE JOY OF HEALTH
A Doctor's Guide to Nutrition and
Alternative Medicine
by Zoltan P. Rona M.D., M.Sc.

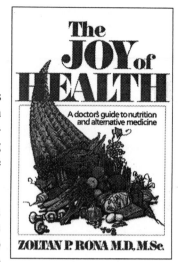

Finally, a medical doctor objectively explores the benefits and pitfalls of alternative health care, based on exceptional nutritional scholarship, long clinical practice, and wide-ranging interactions with "established" and alternative practitioners throughout North America.

The Joy of Health is must reading before you seek the advice of an alternative health care provider. Can a chiropractor or naturopath help your condition? What are viable alternatives to standard cancer care? Is Candida a real disease? Can you really extend your life with megavitamins? Might hidden food allergies be the root of many physical and emotional problems?

- Get clear-cut answers to the most commonly asked questions about nutrition and preventive medicine
- Explore various treatments for 47 conditions and diseases
- Make informed choices about food, diets and supplements
- Discover startling information about food allergies and related conditions
- Explore 20 different types of diets and recipes
- Cut through advertising claims and vested-interest scare tactics
- Empower yourself to achieve a high level of wellness

0-87542-684-0, 264 pgs., 6 x 9, softcover   **$12.95**

Prices subject to change without notice.

KUNDALINI AND THE CHAKRAS
A Practical Manual—Evolution in this Lifetime
by Genevieve Paulson

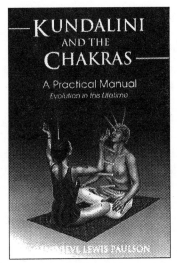

The mysteries of Kundalini revealed! We all possess the powerful evolutionary force of Kundalini that can open us to genius states, psychic powers and cosmic consciousness. As the energies of the Aquarian Age intensify, more and more people are experiencing the "big release" spontaneously but have been ill-equipped to channel its force in a productive manner. This book shows you how to release Kundalini gradually and safely, and is your guide to sating the strange, new appetites which result when life-in-process "blows open" your body's many energy centers.

The section on chakras brings new understanding to these "dials" on our life machine (body). It is the most comprehensive information available for cleansing and developing the chakras and their energies. Read *Kundalini and the Chakras* and prepare to make a quantum leap in your spiritual growth!

0-87542-592-5, 224 pgs. 6 x 9, illus., color plates, softcover $14.95

ENERGIZE!
The Alchemy of Breath & Movement
for Health & Transformation
by Elrond, Juliana and Sophia Blawyn
and Suzanne Jones

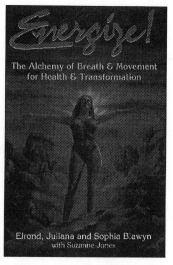

Meeting the needs of our daily obligations can drain us, frustrate us, and slowly kill us in both body and spirit. If you wish to pursue spiritual growth and you lack the strength to devote to this goal, this book can help. With just a few minutes a day of dynamic movement and consciously controlled breathing, you will begin to move your Chi, or vital energy, and you will experience heightened levels of physical energy, greater mental clarity, and a more fit and flexible body. As your reservoir of energy increases, your joy in life will increase, you will possess a greater capacity to function happily and productively in your daily life, and your spiritual progress begins.

Energize! blends the esoteric traditions of yoga, sufism and taoism. You have the remarkable opportunity to learn Chinese *T'ai Chi Chi Kung, T'ai Chi Ruler,* and Red Dragon *Chi Kung*; East Indian Chakra Energizers; Middle Eastern Sufi Earth Dancing, Veil Dancing and Whirling; and the Native American Dance of the Four Directions, all at your own pace in the privacy of your own home.

0-87542-060-5, 240 pgs., 6 x 9, 96 illus., softcover   **$10.00**

AWAKENING THE LIFE FORCE
the Philosophy & Psychology of "Spontaneous Yoga"
by Rajarshi Muni

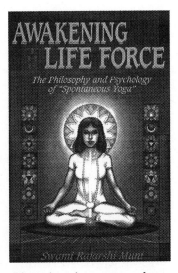

This book is about higher yoga—not physical exercises or meditation to achieve inner peace and happiness (though these may be its by-products or used in preparation for higher yoga). *Awakening the Life Force* is about a proven process by which you can achieve, eternally, liberation from the limitations of time and space, unlimited divine powers, and an immortal, physically perfect divine body that is retained forever. The sages who composed the ancient scriptures achieved such a state, as have men and women of all religious traditions. How? Through the process of "spontaneous" yoga.

In spontaneous yoga, the body and mind are surrendered to the spontaneous workings of the awakened life force: prana. This awakened prana works in its own amazing way to purify the physical and nonphysical bodies of an individual. Whatever path, religion or teaching you follow, *Awakening the Life Force* can help you understand the fascinating physical and metaphysical cosmos in which you live. It reveals how anyone with genuine sincerity can practice dharma, or pure conscious living, which results in prosperity, pleasure, happiness, and the joy of selflessness.

0-87542-581-X, 224 pgs., 7 x 10, 8 color plates, softcover   **$15.00**

A CHAKRA & KUNDALINI WORK-BOOK

Psycho-Spiritual Techniques for Health, Rejuvenation, Psychic Powers and Spiritual Realization
by Dr. Jonn Mumford (Swami Anandakapila Saraswati)

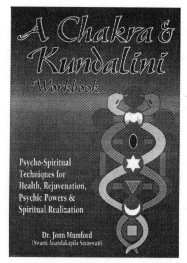

Spend just a few minutes each day on the remarkable psycho-physiological techniques in this book and you will quickly build a solid experience of drugless inner relaxation that will lead towards better health, a longer life, and greater control over your personal destiny. Furthermore, you will lay a firm foundation for the subsequent chapters leading to the attainment of super-normal powers (i.e., photographic memory, self-anesthesia and mental calculations), an enriched Inner Life, and ultimate transcendence. Learn techniques to use for burn-out, mild to moderate depression, insomnia, general anxiety and panic attacks, and reduction of mild to moderate hypertension. Experience sex for consciousness expansion, ESP development, and positive thinking. The text is supplemented with tables and illustrations to bridge the distance from information to personal understanding. In addition, the author has added a simple outline of a 12-week practice schedule referenced directly back to the first nine chapters.

A Chakra & Kundalini Workbook is one of the clearest, most approachable books on Yoga there is. Tailored for the Western mind, this is a practical system of personal training suited for anyone in today's active and complex world.

1-56718-473-1, 296 pgs., 7 x 10, 8 color plates, softcover   **$16.95**